Acrodermatitis Enteropathica

Pooya Khan Mohammad Beigi
Emanual Maverakis

Acrodermatitis Enteropathica

A Clinician's Guide

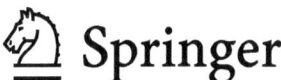 Springer

Pooya Khan Mohammad Beigi, Msc, MD
University of British Columbia
Vancouver
British Columbia
Canada

New York Medical College
Valhalla
NY
USA

Emanual Maverakis, MD
University of California Davis
Sacramento
CA
USA

ISBN 978-3-319-17818-9   ISBN 978-3-319-17819-6   (eBook)
DOI 10.1007/978-3-319-17819-6

Library of Congress Control Number: 2015944512

Springer Cham Heidelberg New York Dordrecht London

Printed on acid-free paper

Springer International Publishing AG Switzerland is part of Springer Science+Business Media (www.springer.com)

To my father,
the best hero of my life,
Mohammad
Khanmohammad Beigi
and
To my mom,
the best queen of my life,
Parvin Mojabi

Preface

When first approached by Dr. Pooya with his original manuscript, I was impressed by his detailed description of numerous case studies of older long-term survivors with chronic, late-diagnosed *acrodermatitis enteropathica* (AE). These cases are not a focus of the book that has evolved subsequently which is regrettable as they did provide an interesting reminder of a clinical presentation of AE which is not always recognized and that the presentation or, at least, the diagnosis may occur over a wide age range. This variation in age of apparent onset is but one of many variations in the clinical presentation of AE attributable primarily to multiple polymorphisms of the SLC39A4 gene.

This book has evolved into a much more comprehensive review including a history of the recognition of our understanding of AE; an up-to-date review of Zn transporters, abnormalities of which are central to the etiology of zinc deficiency. The attention directed to the genetics of this disorder is very useful, as is the clinical description of cases treated at the Razi Hospital in Iran over a relatively short time period which provides some indication of the variation in clinical presentation.

To a clinician, the outstanding good fortune about AE is that ever since Moynihan's observation [1], there has been a reliable and dramatically effective treatment for this erstwhile, often fatal, disease by early childhood. Prior to the observation of the efficacy of Zn, a number of remedies, or rather partial remedies, had been reported, most notably the value of diiodohydroxyquin in some but not all patients. Observation of the potential usefulness of this treatment was serendipitous, and the reason for its partial success remains a matter of conjecture. In contrast, with confirmation of Moynihan's observation on the efficacy of generous Zn supplements, including our own research in Denver [2–5], it rapidly became apparent in the early mid-1970s that AE is an inherited disease of Zn deficiency that could be "cured" by administering larger quantities of Zn than those normally required and that relapse could be prevented by lifelong administration of frequent, if not daily, Zn supplements. Moreover, this supplement is effective when taken orally, a fact that will be discussed further below. Together with the dramatic skin lesions which should alert the clinician to the possibility of AE and, with possible exceptions, ease of confirmation of the diagnosis with a plasma Zn measurement, this disease progressed from a puzzling, severe often fatal illness to one that could be treated rapidly and with great satisfaction to the patient and caregiver.

Though described later, a brief synopsis of the clinical features of AE is merited in this preface. The skin lesions are the outstanding, consistent, clinically evident feature of AE. Typically most pronounced around the body orifices, they are also frequently present at the extremities and can be more generalized. The lesions are most commonly an acute, erythematous, vesiculobullous, or pustular dermatitis, but they may also be or progress to chronic hyperkeratotic psoriaform plaques. These lesions typically become manifest in early to mid-infancy, but are delayed if breast-fed. The other two features quoted as typical of AE are alopecia and diarrhea, neither of which is a constant finding, though variable gastrointestinal symptoms are usually present at diagnosis. The untreated case typically has a downhill course with progressive growth failure, frequent infections associated with multiple defects in the immune system, and, in the pre-Zn era, often ending fatally in early childhood. Very frequent, probable consistent features were psychological disorders which can include lethargy, anorexia, loss of hedonic tone, or overt depression. As with skin lesions, the response to Zn supplementation is apparent within 2–3 days of starting, illustrating the importance of Zn for function of the central nervous system. Relatively little detailed attention was directed to the typical growth failure. No details were recorded <5 %, but this appears to have been primarily linear growth failure except for cases that had a fatal outcome in which wasting was also likely to be evident. The linear growth failure is not without interest, given the recognized need for Zn for epiphyseal growth and the extreme skeletal deformities observed in large mammals which were zinc depleted. This early evidence of the importance of Zn for linear growth is of greater recognized importance today, when the short and later associated adverse effects of stunting are clearly recognized.

This preface includes an overview of four AE patients shared by me, a pediatrician, and my colleague Dr Neldner, a dermatologist at the time when Dr Moynihan's report quickly aroused our interest in utilizing the resources of my micronutrient laboratory at the University of Colorado School of Medicine. This was an exciting time for us when there was a strong need to confirm the apparent likelihood that AE was a genetically determined disease of Zn deficiency.

In no particular order, the first subject presented to us as a boy aged 31 months who developed classical skin lesions at the age of 6 weeks while fed with a cow milk formula. Diiodohydroxyquin was ineffective, poorly tolerated, and discontinued. At that time he had skin lesions, total alopecia, and diarrhea. He was commenced on expressed breast milk, increasing to 60 oz/day, and had total clinical remission and was only troubled with intermittent skin lesions and behavioral change until age 31 months when he was first seen by us and started on Zn. He remained in full remission on Zn and only had a temporary recurrence when he discontinued his Zn supplements as an adolescent. The reason for the favorable response to expressed breast milk remains unexplained. This milk will not have a high concentration of Zn, and the favorable efficiency of Zn absorption from breast milk appears to be explicable on the basis of this low concentration. However, the large quantities of the milk given in this case could have resulted in a relatively high intake of Zn.

Subject 2 found us at the age of 37 months. She was breast-fed for 4 months and progressed well. Three weeks after switching to formula, however, the typical and severe AE skin rash developed; hair growth was very poor; she became very irritable and anorectic and had growth failure. She had a very good response to diiodohydroxyquin, but linear growth remained poor. Skin lesions reappeared when diiodohydroxyquin was discontinued for 2 weeks when first seen by us. She was then started on $ZnSO_4.7H_2O$ 50 mg × 2 daily (a little over 20 mg Zn/day). This was followed by rapid disappearance of all skin lesions and catch-up growth. Her mother was most impressed, however, with her improvement in hedonic tone. Apparently her daughter had never been seen to smile, but within 1–2 days of starting Zn, she was laughing and overtly happy. We have continued to informally follow this case for nearly 40 years. She has normal growth and has done very well academically, working in the health system, with two normal pregnancies resulting in two very healthy adolescent children. She does, as expected, need to continue her Zn-sulfate, which for many years has required 225 mg/day (~40 mg Zn) which has had no adverse effect on copper status.

The third subject was a girl aged 12 years and 11 months who developed a rash on the face, followed by the scalp, hands, and feet at the age of 3 months. Three weeks later, vomiting and diarrhea commenced, and she became dehydrated. The response to diiodohydroxyquin was disappointing, though diarrhea ceased at age 11 months and she did survive. When referred to us at 12 years, she had multiple hyperkeratotic, mildly erythematous patches on the hands, forearms, elbows, axillae, knees, ankles, feet, and perineum. The nails were deformed and atrophic with paronychia on fingers and toes. Cheilosis was evident at the corner of her mouth, and her tongue was lumpy and scarred. Hair growth was poor. Photophobia was severe with a punctate keratopathy of both eyes and blepharitis of both eyelids. She was stunted with a bone age of 10 years. She was depressed with little communication. Zn therapy was started at a dose of 50 mg $ZnSO_4.7H_2O \times 4$ daily reducing to $\times 3$ daily after 2 weeks. Her long-term skin lesions started to improve 2 days after commencement of the Zn supplement, but took 2 months for these chronic lesions to disappear. During this period she had become more active, communicative, and cheerful. Her eye lesions had improved. Our experience with this subject demonstrated that even chronic lesions of AE at an older age will respond to Zn supplementation. She also illustrates the variety of organs that can be affected by AE.

Our fourth subject was an adult woman aged 23 years, a long-term patient of Dr Neldner's, who had developed signs of the disorder at age 1 and 3 months and was "near death" at age 1.5 years at which point she responded favorably to diiodohydroxyquin but remained reclusive and depressed. Two pregnancies resulted in spontaneous abortion, and she delivered one anencephalic stillbirth, reminiscent of a congenital malformation observed in zinc-depleted mice [6].

Three of these four subjects had hypozincemia prior to Zn therapy which normalized rapidly with therapy. Subject 1 while on breast milk had a level of 64 ug/dL; Subject 2 had a level of 44 ug/dL while on diiodohydroxyquin. Plasma Zn in Subject 3 was 30 ug/dL before Zn therapy. Subject 4 had a plasma Zn of 39 ug/dL when without skin lesions on diiodohydroxyquin. When the later was withheld, a clinical exacerbation occurred after 8 days, starting with aphthous ulceration, quickly involving the skin, paronychia, and depression. There was rapid remission with $ZnSO_4.7H_2O$ at 220 mg $\times 3$ daily. There was rapid clinical remission, and Zn therapy was discontinued after 10 days. Remission continued for 5 weeks at which time her plasma Zn had fallen to <20ug/g. Diiodohydroxyquin was ineffective in achieving a remission or a normal plasma Zn, both of which were then achieved long term with 50 mg ZnSO4.7H2O $\times 2$ daily.

Numerous cases of classical or possible AE have been referred subsequently, but typically pediatricians now treat with Zn without further referral after hypozincemia is confirmed.

These subjects contribute to our understanding of the diversity of the clinical features of AE, the characteristic skin lesions being the only clinical manifestation which should ensure that consideration of this disease is high in the differential diagnosis. At that "early time," the clinical research directed to these subjects provided very strong support for the conclusion that AE is a disease attributable to severe Zn deficiency, which can be treated and clinical remission maintained with quantities of Zn higher than those normally required to meet physiological requirements for this essential trace mineral.

In addition to the outstanding and quickly indisputable impact that generous Zn supplements, if maintained, provided a clinical cure for AE, this discovery has advanced our understanding of Zn metabolism and homeostasis. The opportunity to do this came some 20 years later with the recognition of the multiple roles of newly discovered Zn transporters in maintaining Zn homeostasis within the cell and within the whole body. These Zn transporters belong to the ZIP and ZnT families. Several of these are known to act in synchrony to regulate Zn absorption into the enterocytes, especially of the duodenum and jejunum, then across these cells and exiting through the basolateral membrane into the portal circulation. Special attention has been given to ZIP4 located at the apical surface of the enterocyte. Evidences from experimental animals support its role in the regulation of absorption of Zn by decreasing the transcription of the SLC39A4 gene when bioavailable Zn in the gut lumen is excessive and increasing the number of ZIP4 transporters when the available Zn in the gut lumen is inadequate [7]. In AE, ZIP4 transporters at the apical surface of the enterocyte are absent or dysfunctional which readily explains the development of severe Zn deficiency in early to mid-infancy when limited Zn stores acquired by the fetus in utero have been fully utilized.

At this time even in experimental animals, evidence for the upregulation of Zn absorption by increasing the number of apical ZIP4 transporters when Zn intake on the apical surface of enterocytes is restricted is limited. With AE, the apical ZIP4 transporters are distorted and in classical severe cases are completely nonfunctional. The phenotype, including plasma Zn in untreated cases, gives irrefutable evidence of the central importance of mucosal surface ZIP4 in active absorption of physiological quantities of Zn by the enterocyte.

Why then are the clinical effects ameliorated and plasma Zn normalized with the administration of quantities of Zn which, especially in young children, are greatly in excess of normal physiological requirements? The answer may lie in the presence of a second passive pathway for Zn absorption through the enterocyte. The existence of this pathway in experimental animals was hypothesized by several investigators in the last century who concluded that their experimental findings could only be explained by the existence of this second pathway [8]. This pathway is linear with a relatively low slope for Zn absorption versus intake. However, at higher, nonphysiological levels of bioavailable Zn, Zn absorption via this pathway, about which relatively little is known, will eventually result in adequate Zn absorption independently of any Zn absorbed via the active pathway. The AE phenotype before and during Zn supplementation is consistent with this conclusion.

References

1. Moynahan EJ. Letter: acrodermatitis enteropathica: a lethal inherited human zinc-deficiency disorder. Lancet. 1974;2(7877):399–400.
2. Neldner KH, Hambidge KM. Zinc therapy of acrodermatitis enteropathica. N Engl J Med. 1975;292(17):879–82.
3. Hambidge KM, Walravens PA, Neldner KH. Zinc and acrodermatitis enteropathica. In: Hambidge KM, Nichols BL, editors. Zinc and copper in clinical medicine. New York: Spectrum Publications, Inc.; 1977. p. 81–98.
4. Hambidge KM. Use of static-argon atmosphere in emission spectrochemical determination of chromium in biological materials. Anal Chem. 1971;43(1):103–7.
5. Walravens PA, Hambidge KM, Neldner KH, Silverman A, van Doorninck WJ, Mierau G, et al. Zinc metabolism in acrodermatitis enteropathica. J Pediatr. 1978;93(1):71–3.

6. Hambidge KM, Neldner KH, Walravens PA. Zinc, acrodermatitis enteropathica and congenital malformations. Lancet. 1975;1:577.
7. Cousins RJ, Liuzzi JP, Lichten LA. Mammalian zinc transport, trafficking, and signals. J Biological Chem. 2006;281(34):24085–9.
8. Lonnerdal B. Intestinal absorption of zinc. In: Mills C, editor. Zinc in Human Biology. Berlin: Springer; 1989. p. 33–55.

K. Michael Hambidge

Acknowledgements

Special Thanks to:

Fatemeh Jalalian
Masoud Beigi, MD
Maryam Beigi
Anthony P. Cheung, MD
Majid Doroudi, PhD
Ladan Fazli, MD
Yahya Dowlati, MD
Amirhosein Emami, MD
Shahin Akhondzadeh, MD
Nafiseh Esmaeili, MD
Amirhoushang Ehsani, MD
Farshad Farnaghi, MD
Kamran Balighi, MD
Minoo Mohraz, MD
Batool Rashidi, MD
Mostafa Shareei, PharmD
Koroush Faghih Nasiri
Arasteh Bidarbakht
Mona Maleki
Negin Askari
Ava Bidgoli

Contents

Contributors

Pooya Khan Mohammad Beigi, MSc, MD University of British Columbia, Vancouver, BC, Canada

New York Medical College, Valhalla, NY, USA

The only main Author of all Chapters and Parts

Emanual Maverakis, MD University of California Davis, Davis, CA, USA

Coauthor in: Sects. 2.2, 3.1, 3.2, all of the Sects. 5.1, 5.2, 5.3, 5.4, 5.5, 5.6, 6, and 7.1, 7.2, 7.3, 7.4, 7.5 and 7.6 as well as Sect. 7.11

Hassan Seirafi, MD Tehran University of Medical Sciences, Tehran, Iran

Coauthor in: Part III and Part IV

Seyed Sajad Niyyati University of British Columbia, Vancouver, BC, Canada

Coauthor in: Part I and II

Michael Hambidge, MD, ScD University of Colorado Denver, Denver, CO, USA

Coauthor in: Preface

Reason Wilken, MD University of California Davis, Davis, CA, USA

Coauthor in: Sects. 2.2, 3.1, 3.2, all of the Sects. 5.1, 5.2, 5.3, 5.4, 5.5, 5.6, 6, and 7.1, 7.2, 7.3, 7.4, 7.5 and 7.6 as well as Sect. 7.11

Sébastien Kury, MD CHU de Nantes Hôtel-Dieu, Service de Génétique Médicale, Nantes, France

Coauthor in: Part I-Sects. 2 and 5

Part I
Overview of Disorder

Chapter 1
History of Acrodermatitis Enteropathica

Acrodermatitis Enteropathica (AE) is an inherited autosomal recessive disorder which often presents in newborn infants [1]. This medical condition occurs as a result of mutation of a zinc transporter that affects the uptake of zinc in the intestine causing a decrease in the level of this elemental mineral in the blood [2]. Prior to this knowledge, untreated AE was considered deleterious to the infant's health and sometimes even fatal [3, 4]. Today however, the treatment involves adding zinc supplements to the patient's diet which can easily improve the condition [1, 3].

Except for the characteristic dermatitis, the symptoms of this disorder vary with age of the patient. Severe uncontrollable diarrhea, mood changes, anorexia, and neurological disorders are frequently reported in infants. Growth retardation, alopecia, weight loss, and recurrent infections have also been reported in toddlers and young children; and spontaneous remission may happen in adolescence [3]. Moreover, there have also been reports of mild sporadic cases in which the patient suffered from ophthalmic, hepatic, and encephalic complications [5]. Interestingly, the signs and symptoms of acquired zinc deficiency include dermatitis on hands and feet, alopecia, diarrhea, and the appearance of inflammatory rashes on the skin of face, hands, feet, and genitals, all of which represent the signs of AE [3].

The disorder was first discovered in 1902 by Wende [5], and further analyzed in 1936 by Brandt [6]. In 1942, it was

P. Khan Mohammad Beigi, E. Maverakis,
Acrodermatitis Enteropathica: A Clinician's Guide,
DOI 10.1007/978-3-319-17819-6_1,
© Springer International Publishing Switzerland 2015

labelled as Acrodermatitis Enteropathica (AE) by Danbolt and Closs, who proposed a clinical definition for AE, based on a triad of pathognomonic symptoms composed by acral and periorifical dermatitis, alopecia, and diarrhea [7]. Subsequently, in 1953 Neldner et al. reported a successful treatment of AE by diiodohydroxyquin, which was consumed orally in order to slow the progress of the disease in children and to prevent fatality in different stages of the disorder [8]. In 1974, Moynahan concluded that AE appeared in patients who suffer from zinc deficiency and that it could be abolished by oral zinc supplementation [9]. Prior to this finding, antibiotic amphotericin B, which increases intestinal membrane permeability to divalent cations, was used to treat the symptoms of this disorder [10].

Moynahan suggested that the absence of an enzyme called oligopeptidase in the intestine was responsible for the decreased serum zinc levels observed in AE patients [9]. Oligopeptidase is secreted by enterocytes for the degradation of proteins and Moynahan proposed that its absence resulted in the accumulation of oligopeptides which then would chelate with zinc, reducing available zinc for absorption. During the 1980s, it was suggested that zinc was mainly absorbed in the duodenum by binding with a low molecular weight zinc-binding ligand, which is mainly secreted by the pancreas and also present in small amounts in breast milk because infants are not capable of ZBL production during early infancy [11, 12]. Recently, it was revealed that the zinc-binding ligand does in fact facilitate zinc absorption [12]; however its mechanism is unknown and its main role in zinc absorption still needs to be elucidated.

In 2002 two independent studies showed that AE was due to homozygous or compound heterozygous mutations of *SLC39A4*, a gene located on chromosomal region 8q24.3, which codes for the zinc-specific transporter ZIP4 (or hZIP4) [13, 14]. This transporter is found more especially in the distal duodenal and proximal jejunal parts of the small [13], where it enables the absorption of zinc from the intestinal lumen. Through its function and localization, ZIP4 plays a major role in human zinc homeostasis, which explains the broad clinical picture of acrodermatitis enteropathica.

References

1. Maverakis E, et al. Acrodermatitis enteropathica and an overview of zinc metabolism. J Am Acad Dermatol. 2007;56(1): 116–24.
2. Puri N. A study of efficacy of oral zinc therapy for acrodermatitis enteropathica. Nasza dermatolologia online. 2013;4:162–6.
3. Van Wouwe JP. Clinical and laboratory diagnosis of acrodermatitis enteropathica. Eur J Pediatr. 1989;149(1):2–8.
4. Aggett PJ. Acrodermatitis enteropathica. J Inherit Metab Dis. 1983;6 Suppl 1:39–43.
5. Wende GW. Epidermolysis bullosa hereditaria. J Cut Dis. 1902;20:537–47.
6. Brandt T. Dermatitis in children with disturbances of the general condition and the absorption of food elements. Acta Derm. 1936;17:513–46.
7. Danbolt N, Closs K. Acrodermatitis enteropathica. Acta Derm Venerol. 1942;23:127–69.
8. Neldner KH, Hambidge KM. Zinc therapy of acrodermatitis enteropathica. N Engl J Med. 1975;292(17):879–82.
9. Moynahan EJ. Letter: acrodermatitis enteropathica: a lethal inherited human zinc-deficiency disorder. Lancet. 1974;2(7877):399–400.
10. Aggett PJ, et al. The therapeutic effect of amphotericin in acrodermatitis enteropathica: hypothesis and implications. Eur J Pediatr. 1981;137(1):23–5.
11. Hurley LS, et al. Zinc-binding ligands in milk and intestine: a role in neonatal nutrition? Proc Natl Acad Sci U S A. 1977;74(8): 3547–9.
12. Evans GW, Johnson PE. Characterization and quantitation of a zinc-binding ligand in human milk. Pediatr Res. 1980;14(7): 876–80.
13. Küry S, et al. Identification of SLC39A4, a gene involved in acrodermatitis enteropathica. Nat Genet. 2002;31(3):239–40.
14. Wang K, et al. Homozygosity mapping places the acrodermatitis enteropathica gene on chromosomal region 8q24.3. Am J Hum Genet. 2001;68(4):1055–60.

Chapter 2
Epidemiology and Etiology

2.1 Epidemiology

AE is not specific to any ethnic population, as cases have been reported from all around the world [1]. It is globally widespread with an estimated incidence of 1 in 500,000 children [1–4]. According to the cases reported in the literature, its prevalence seems higher in populations from the Mediterranean basin, probably because of their relatively high overall consanguinity [3]. There is also no gender predilection observed in AE [1, 3]. Compared to the United States, the diagnosis of AE may be more difficult in developing countries where dietary zinc deficiencies are quite common, a problem emphasized in the World Health Report 2002 [5]. Approximately two billion individuals may be zinc deficient in these regions of the world [6], where infants and children are the most affected. The regions particularly affected by zinc deficiency problems include Southeast Asia and sub-Saharan Africa, since about 40 % of their preschool children have been reported to have zinc-related growth problems [7]. It has been reported that moderate zinc deficiency affects approximately 3 % of adolescents in rural areas of Middle East and North Africa [8]. Correcting this situation would have dramatic impacts on the morbidity and mortality of young children and modest effects on their growth. However, it is important to tackle malnutrition of these regions as a

P. Khan Mohammad Beigi, E. Maverakis,
Acrodermatitis Enteropathica: A Clinician's Guide,
DOI 10.1007/978-3-319-17819-6_2,
© Springer International Publishing Switzerland 2015

whole, instead of undertaking zinc deficiency in isolation. As a result, including zinc in a multiple micronutrient supplementation and promoting their use would be an effective method of dealing with this situation [9].

Even though AE is not as prevalent in the United States as it is in countries with high rates of consanguinity, acquired zinc deficiency has been reported in American newborns and children. There have been several studies that reported of American infants having exceptionally low hair and plasma zinc levels [10]. Deficiency in zinc, may have serious and permanent growth and developmental effects on children and infants of which some were reported in a study from Denver in 1972 where some of the children with zinc deficiency also suffered from growth retardation [11]. The main contributing factors resulting in infant zinc deficiency in the United States include popular infant milk formulae having low zinc concentration and the necessity of large amounts of zinc for infant rapid growth [12].

Lactation, alcoholism, old age, and metabolic disorders are associated with zinc deficiency in the American adult demographic [8]. A recent study found that about 30 % of pregnant women of low socioeconomic status had low body zinc levels. Insufficient maternal zinc levels could have severe effects on prenatal growth and development of the child, such as congenital malformation of the central nervous system [12]. In the light of this, more research and attention should be devoted to increasing knowledge, raising awareness, and correction of these nutritional problems.

2.2   Etiology

2.2.1   Molecular Etiology of AE

Presently, AE is considered a treatable disorder since it can be simply managed with zinc supplementation once diagnosed. As a result of the profound effects this disease has on human physiology, which are particularly pronounced in infants, medical science still considers it as one of the most intriguing and interesting disorders. AE is suggested to have an autosomal recessive mode of inheritance by genealogic data [13].

AE presents a multitude of opportunities for research; however, at present only rare cases are referred to academic medical centers since this disorder is easily treatable. Consequently, the study of this disorder is rarely done. Two main hypotheses are proposed. One is based on a problem of zinc bioavailability and the other on an intrinsic defect of zinc transport by the affected individual.

2.2.2 Hypothetical Etiology 1: The Alteration of Zinc Bioavailability

As patients with AE can obtain only a small amount of zinc through dietary sources, supplementing the diet with sufficient amounts of zinc can raise the level of zinc in blood plasma to a normal level and result in the resolution of the disorder. Although the amount of zinc in breast milk and infant formula are roughly equal, the zinc in breast milk has been observed to be more absorbable by infants with AE and this phenomenon has become an interesting matter among dermatologists, pediatricians, and medical researchers [14].

To date, research has indicated that the zinc absorption process is very complex. Research laboratory results illustrate that the zinc binding ligand found in human milk facilitates zinc absorption in the intestine and the ligand's presence results in high bioavailability of zinc in human milk [15] (Fig. 2.1).

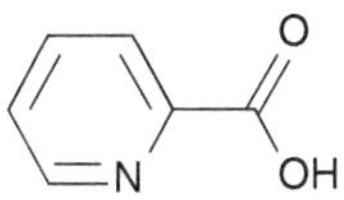

Figure 2.1 Molecular structure of picolinic acid

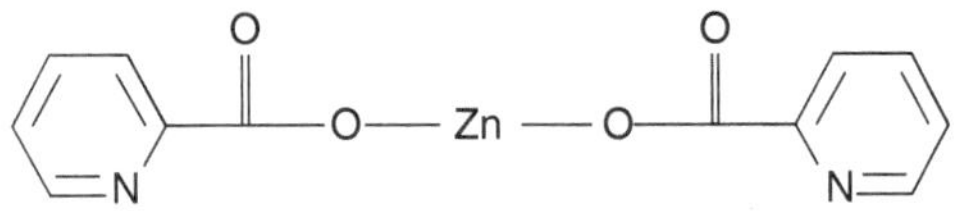

FIGURE 2.2 Molecular structure of zinc picolinate (zinc bound pico-linic acid)

Evans and Johnson found the concentration of picolinic acid, a zinc binding ligand, in human milk to be much higher than that in either bovine milk or infant formulas. The higher concentration of picolinic acid in human milk could result in the formation of additional zinc picolinate complexes which would be more absorbable by the intestine compared to ionic zinc or zinc complexed with other ligands [15]. Conversely, Rebello et al. found the amount of picolinic acid present in human pancreatic juice or intestine to be less than 2.5 µM. They also found the amount of picolinic acid present in human milk to be approximately 3.7 µM and declared it insignificant in zinc absorption due to its minimal quantity. Rebello et al. also emphasized that they cannot explain the inordinately high values of picolinic acid reported by Evans and Johnson [16]. Later on, it was discovered that supplementation of picolinic acid only increases zinc turnover without increasing retention since its administration to individuals only increased zinc excretion, which would lead to zinc depletion in the absence of adequate zinc supplementation [17, 18] (Fig. 2.2).

Eckhert et al. discovered that alongside elemental zinc, breast milk contains a protein zinc-binding ligand with a low molecular weight of about 10,000 Da, while the ligand along-side elemental zinc observed in bovine milk has a greater molecular weight. The ligand present in bovine milk does not improve zinc absorption; as a result AE symptoms often appear when the infants' diet is switched to bovine milk [19].

Casey, Walravens, et al. were able to find protein zinc-binding ligands in the duodenum with the same properties of the ligand described above, in pancreatic secretions and they also confirmed that the weight of the ZBL is significant for its function [20]. Recently, researchers have hypothesized that AE may be caused by a mutation in the gene *SLC39A4* coding for the hZip4 Zn transporter present in intestinal cells of the intestine [3, 4]. This hypothesis is supported by studies that have concluded that AE patients and healthy individuals have similar duodenal ZBL secretions or that the amount of ZBL present in the intestine is insignificant in zinc absorption [16, 21].

Following the acknowledgment that this zinc deficiency condition is a disorder, the main concern of medical researchers has been the discovery of the mechanism for zinc absorption from a regular diet: a mechanism that seems to function insufficiently in AE patients. Interestingly, Casey et al. determined that zinc absorption was decreased in patients with AE compared to individuals in the control group, even though both groups had the same amount of ZBL present in their duodenal secretion [21]. At the time, it was concluded that ZBL in duodenal secretion of AE patients did not function sufficiently, which could be due to their abnormal nature as a result of the AE disorder [21]. Moreover, an alternative hypothesis is that since zinc absorption was decreased in AE patients, while both groups (AE patients and control group) had similar duodenal ZBL secretions, the insufficient zinc absorption may be due to malfunction of the zinc transporters present in apical intestinal cells, impairing the uptake of zinc [3, 21]. This hypothesis will be discussed later in this section.

Cousins and Smith noticed that only 10 % of the zinc in fat-free breast milk was accompanied by the ZBL that has the low molecular weight; when more zinc was added in vitro to the breast milk, almost all the zinc became ZBL bound [22]. Lonnerdal's research indicated that an increase in the amount of dietary protein led to an increase in zinc absorption in a linear fashion, which may have been as a result of amino acids released from the protein keeping the zinc in solution and increasing bioavailability of the zinc [23–25]. Amino acids such as histidine and methionine as well as EDTA, a low molecular weight ion, and organic acids have been known to boost zinc absorption and have been used for zinc supplements [23]. For instance, clinical studies have shown histidine to have a positive effect on zinc absorption since it is a good chelator of zinc [26]. It is important to note that high doses of histidine were reported to enhance urinary excretion of zinc, hence the molar ratio of histidine to zinc is of importance when considering the administration of histidine to zinc deficient patients [27]. It was also found in a clinical study that infants who were fed formula with a high protein concentration had lower plasma zinc concentrations than infants fed formula with less protein [28]. On the other hand, zinc found in infant formula was observed to be more absorbable compared to bovine milk, which could be due to the inhibitory effect of casein that is present in bovine milk on zinc absorption [25]. This could be caused by phosphorylated serine and threonine residues on partially undigested casein subunits that bind zinc and reduce zinc bioavailability [29, 30]. Interestingly in a recent study, it was found that casein phosphopeptides (CPP) added to a phytate-containing solution significantly increased calcium and zinc absorption in suckling rat pups as well as in human intestinal cells (Caco-2) in culture [31]. A human study showed that CPP addition to a high phytate meal had no effect on zinc absorption, as a result the effect of CPP may be dependent on the phytate content of the meal [32].

Menard and Cousins have noted that the zinc found in the intestine tends to be bound to citrate, which has a molecular weight of 600–650 Da [33]. This zinc-citrate compound is part of the ZBL mentioned previously; however research has indicated that the presence of citrate as part of the ligand complex does not enhance the absorption of zinc in the rat intestine [34].

Due to the significant interest of medical researchers concerning ZBL, there have been many research reports in this area. However, the exact role of ZBL in zinc absorption is yet to be elucidated. Sang et al. stated that prostaglandin E2 facilitates zinc absorption in the intestine [35]. Furthermore, the total amount of zinc present in the human body was seen to have an effect on its absorption. For instance, in an individual with low levels of zinc, zinc absorption is more widespread and would occur at a higher rate compared to cases where the amount of zinc present in the body was sufficient or more than the required amount [23].

Other factors such as the presence of iron, cadmium, low-molecular-weight ligands, and chelators also affect zinc absorption [23]. For instance, when adult individuals were administered high doses of inorganic iron in solution, there was a decrease in zinc absorption as plasma levels of zinc were seen to diminish [23, 36]. But when the administered solution also contained ZBL, zinc absorption was unaffected. It is likely that the inhibitory effect occurs only when iron-to-zinc ratio is very high and is in solution. When the same amount of high dose iron was administered to adult individuals as supplement tablets, no inhibitory effect on zinc absorption was observed; which suggested that only iron in solution can affect zinc absorption [23]. Interestingly, when infants were fed iron drops (30 mg/drop), zinc absorption was also unaltered [37]. This suggests that iron supplementation does not affect zinc absorption and if iron and zinc supplements are administered apart from meals, an inhibitory effect will be found only when the iron-to-zinc ratio is very high [23].

Furthermore, nontoxic levels of cadmium were seen to have no effect on zinc absorption. Since zinc can form a complex with low-molecular-weight ligands or chelators, such as ZBL, an increase in levels of ligands or chelators were observed to have a positive effect on zinc absorption. Moreover, amino acids like histidine that are good chelators of zinc can increase zinc absorption in the intestine; however, very high levels of histidine often result in excess urinary excretion of zinc and decrease in plasma zinc levels [23].

2.2.3 Hypothetical Etiology 2: A Defective Zinc Transporter

This second hypothesis is supported notably by arguments against a problem of zinc bioavailability. At least two studies had indeed concluded that AE patients and healthy individuals had similar duodenal ZBL secretions or that the amount of ZBL present in the intestine was insignificant in zinc absorption [16, 21]. If the problem in AE patients did not relate to zinc consumption itself, then it could be due to a defect in the molecular protein ensuring its absorption from the intestinal lumen.

Cloning of the first human zinc-specific transporters is quite recent, as ZnT-1 (*SLC30A1*) and ZnT-2 (*SLC30A2*) were identified in 1995 [38] and 1966 [39], respectively. In 1997, as they were working on a mouse model of pallid mutant, Huang and Gitschier serendipitously found that homozygous mutations of ZnT-4 (*SLC30A4*) caused the *lethal milk* phenotype in the strain they were studying [40]. Interestingly, *lethal milk,* which is a recessive condition, could be considered as the murine counterpart of human AE, keeping in mind that the consequence of biallelic ZnT-4 mutations are not seen in the mutant mouse herself, but in her suckling offspring. Mutations of ZnT-4 entail a decrease in milk zinc levels of *lethal milk* mothers, which result in a generalized zinc deficiency and eventually death of the suckling pups.

Yet, *SLC30A4* turned out not to have any link with AE, as its involvement in the disease was ruled out by sequencing in AE families [41]. Several other candidates were discarded this way, including ZnT-1 to ZnT-3 (Küry et al., unpublished data) and ZnT-5 (aka hZTL1 or *SLC30A5*) [42], until Wang et al. highlighted a susceptibility locus for AE on 8q24.3 [43]. Within this locus, two independent teams cloned the gene *SLC39A4* [4, 44], presenting a high degree of homology with the ZIP (zinc/iron-like proteins) family of zinc transporters identified several years also in plant and yeast [45–47] and with the three human ZIP family freshly identified [48]. Both teams could establish a relationship between homozygous or compound heterozygous mutations of *SLC39A4* and the symptoms of zinc deficiency in several AE patients originating from Tunisia, France, Egypt and Jordania [4, 44]. Since then, the relationship between AE and mutations of *SLC39A4* was largely confirmed, as more than 40 mutations were reported worldwide that are distributed along the gene [3, 44, 49]. Recommendations on the molecular diagnosis of AE were detailed in a clinical utility gene card [50].

Apart from likely founder effects noted for instance for the Tunisian mutation c.1224_1228del (p.Gly409Leufs*7) [3], mutations are almost always private and no hotspot is observed within the gene. A slight recurrence can however be noted for a few mutations such as c.599C>T (p.Pro200Leu) or c.192 + 19G > A (p.?). The mutations encountered so far are nonsense, missense and splice site mutations or small frame-shift insertions/deletions. No large rearrangement encom-passing one exon or more has ever been reported. All genuine cases of AE have either a homozygous *SLC39A4* mutation or compound *SLC39A4* heterozygous mutations. Beside these cases following a Mendelian autosomal reces-sive mode of inheritance, transient forms of zinc deficiency have also been observed in heterozygous carriers of *SLC39A4* mutations, which would rather follow an autosomal dominant mode of inheritance with incomplete penetrance (Küry et al., unpublished personal observation). The inconsistency of this transient form of zinc deficiency suggests that its occurrence is subjected to the co-existence of an additional risk factors, which might be prematurity, intestinal pathology or a nutri-tional factor decreasing zinc bioavailability.

According to its function, and its expression-, tissue- and cellular-localizations, *SLC39A4* immediately appeared as the ideal candidate for explaining AE. On the one hand, it is highly expressed in the kidney, but most importantly in the duodenal and jejunal parts of the intestinal tract [2, 4], that is to say the main sites of dietary zinc absorption and thereby of human zinc homeostasis. On the other hand, its related pro-tein SLC39A4 (or ZIP4) is localized at the apical membrane of the enterocytes [4], where it transports dietary zinc from the intestinal lumen to the intracellular compartment. Rapidly, functional studies in cellular and murine models showed that SLC39A4 transporter is a key component of a human zinc homeostasis [51] and they confirmed the correla-tion between *SLC39A4* mutations and severe zinc deficiency [52–56]. AE patients' mutations were shown to either dimin-ish the efficiency of zinc transport by SLC39A4, or to induce its mislocalization in the nuclear envelope and endoplasmic reticulum, which could be attributed to the misfolding of the protein and prevention of its proper glycolysation and local-ization [51, 57].

The finding of the molecular cause of acrodermatitis enteropathica gave new insight on the mechanism of intesti-nal zinc absorption. Several studies focused then on SLC39A4, which allowed better comprehension of the overall phenomenon. Thus, the first step for zinc absorption involves the arrival of zinc to the intestine after the food is ingested by the individual and partially digested both mechanically and chemically in the mouth cavity and stomach. Subsequently, as the zinc comes in contact with the apical membrane of the intestinal villous, where the transmembrane protein *SLC39A4* (ZIP4) is located, the zinc is actively transported into the enterocyte from the small intestinal lumen [53]. Research on human cells over-expressing the ZIP4 gene showed increased accumulation of ^{65}Zn, indicating a carrier-mediated uptake process [53]. Moreover, in vivo and in vitro studies have shown that *SLC39A4* undergoes posttranscriptional regulation in response to zinc levels: in zinc-deficient conditions the *SLC39A4* (ZIP4) protein was concentrated on the cell membrane whereas in zinc-replete cells *SLC39A4* was sequestered and mainly found in intracellular compartments [51, 53]. Studies on the mouse homologue of *SLC39A4*, mZIP4, highlighted its control by zinc availability: in zinc deficient conditions, mZIP4 accumulated at the plasma membrane, whereas zinc repletion increased its endocytosis [51, 57]. This mechanism would prevent intracellular accumulation of zinc and thereby from zinc toxicity when dietary zinc amounts are adequate [53]. This responsiveness of SLC39A4 to variations of extracellular zinc conditions is altered by certain AE mutations, which impede the accumulation of the protein during dietary zinc deficiency [57].

2.2.4   Alternative Forms of AE-like Zinc Deficiencies

Interestingly, about half of the patients suspected of having AE have no mutation in coding introns, or promoting sequence of *SLC39A4* [58]. In addition, a few patients with a severe form of zinc deficiency very suggestive of AE exhibit only a heterozygous *SLC39A4* mutation [58]. This suggests either possible alterations of yet unidentified regulating sequences of the *SLC39A4* gene in these patients, or dysregulation of epigenetic mechanisms involving methylation or miRNAs. Alternatively, other zinc transporters might be affected in some cases of acrodermatitis enteropathica [44, 59, 60]. From a semantic point of view, cases of zinc deficiency not caused by homozygous or compound heterozygous mutations of *SLC39A4* are not genuine AE and would rather be labelled as AE-like disorders.

So far, only one form of inherited zinc deficiency alternative to AE has been identified in humans. It is caused by mutations of *SLC30A2* [61], a member of the very same family as *SLC30A4* that is involved in the mouse *lethal milk* phenotype. Incidentally, the transient form of zinc deficiency associated with *SLC30A2* is more similar to mouse *lethal milk* than to human AE. Mutations of the zinc transporter gene induce decreased milk zinc levels in the nursing mother, which are responsible for a lactogenic transient neonatal zinc deficiency (TNZD; MIM#608118) in the exclusively breast-fed baby. TNZD would be inherited according to either autosomal recessive [61, 62] or autosomal dominant [63–65] mode. Zinc transporter *SLC30A2* (or ZNT2), encoded by *SLC30A2*, contributes to the efflux of zinc from cytosol of secreting mammary epithelial cells to milk, by transporting labile zinc from cytoplasm to endosomal vesicles which is then trafficked to the cell membrane and exocytosed to the milk [66].

From the examples of AE and TNZD, one could expect other forms of zinc deficiency related to zinc transporters. Beside *SLC39A4* and *SLC30A2*, human zinc homeostasis is indeed sustained by two zinc transporter families of 10 SLC30 (ZNT) and 14 SLC39 (ZIP) members [67–70], the alteration of which might have impact on body zinc levels. Knock-out mouse models showed that ZNT transporters regulate intracellular zinc concentration by either promoting zinc efflux or zinc transport into intracellular vesicles [71]. In contrast, ZIP transporters ensure the uptake of zinc into cells [72]. Members of the ZNT family have six transmembrane domains with a long histidine loop between transmembrane domains IV and V, which is likely a zinc-binding domain [73, 74].

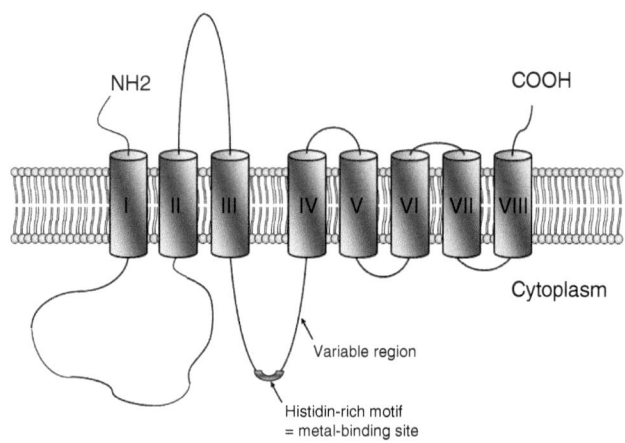

FIGURE 2.3 Predicted structure of ZIP4 protein. The dark grey barrels represent the transmembrane domains. It is characterized by 8 transmembrane domains organized into two blocks of 3 and 5 separated by a histidine-rich cytoplasmic metal-binding site

ZIP family members are characterized by eight transmembrane domains organized into two blocks of three and five domains separated by a histidine-rich cytoplasmic metal-binding site, as seen in Fig. 2.3 [45, 75].

Theoretically, the best ZIP and ZNT candidates for inherited forms of zinc deficiency comparable to AE would be those abundantly present in absorptive enterocytes. According to mouse and various rodent models, a short list of candidate genes can be inferred, which include *SLC30A1*, *SLC30A2*, *SLC30A4*, *SLC30A5*, *SLC30A6*, *SLC30A7*, *SLC39A4*, and *SLC39A5* [76]. In addition, the sole member of GufA subfamily of ZIP family, *SLC39A11*, is also abundantly expressed in murine digestive system, and notably in the stomach, ileum, and caecum [77, 78], which do not constitute the primary intestinal sites of zinc homeostasis, but could have an important role in intestinal zinc absorption. Among these candidates, we note *SLC30A1*, which was the first human zinc transporter to be discovered; beside small intestine, it is highly expressed in renal tubular epithelium, and placenta [79]. Its function is to transfer zinc from enterocytes into circulation [80]. As for *SLC30A2*, it is involved in *lethal milk*; it is highly expressed in the mammary gland, where it is associated with milk-containing vesicles [40, 79]. Contrary to *SLC30A1* and *SLC30A2*, *SLC30A4* is more tissue-specific; it is more abundantly expressed on the apical membrane of enterocytes and it functions to absorb dietary zinc from the intestinal lumen. Interestingly, its expression is regulated in order to maintain intracellular zinc homeostasis. For instance, in a healthy individual, zinc deficiency causes increased expression of ZIP4 whereas zinc supplementation causes decreased expression. It is this transporter that is defective in AE patients [53, 81].

If we seek potential candidate genes for a form of zinc deficiency more like the mouse *lethal milk*, the best ones would be those expressed in the mammary gland, that is to say *SLC30A1*, *SLC30A2*, *SLC30A3* and *SLC39A3* [66]. An extended list would comprise the genes whose encoded zinc transporters are abundant during lactation and would have a major contribution to zinc redistribution in the body, which include *SLC39A3*, *SLC39A5*, *SLC39A7*, *SLC39A8*, *SLC39A10*, *SLC39A11* for ZIP transporter genes and *SLC30A2*, *SLC30A4* and *SLC30A9* for ZNT transporter genes [66].

Another candidate gene for inherited forms of zinc deficiency would be *SLC30A1*. Research has indeed shown that the human ZIP1 protein, expressed in human intestinal Caco-2 cell line derived from epithelial colorectal adenocarcinoma cells, has a major effect on zinc absorption. Localization of this protein depends on the level of maturity of the Caco-2 cell [82]. The ZIP1 protein is located in the proximity of the apical membrane of the intestinal lumen in differentiated Caco-2 cells; while in undifferentiated Caco-2 cells ZIP1 is localized in the endoplasmic reticulum by the means of a protein disulfide isomerase (PDI) marker. As a result, undifferentiated Caco-2 cells are insufficient in zinc absorption [31].

As the ZIP1 is located beneath the intestinal microvilli in differentiated cells but is not present in the apical membrane, it can only affect zinc absorption indirectly. The indirect effect of the ZIP1 protein in zinc absorption is demonstrated by the 20 % reduction in zinc uptake in cells that have had their ZIP1 gene knocked-out. It has been observed that zinc uptake is doubled in cells where the ZIP1 gene is overexpressed [59]. Additionally, there have been other studies in which these results have been duplicated: overexpression of ZIP1 in PC-3 prostate cells [83]. These studies clearly illustrate the role of ZIP1 in absorption of zinc in the intestine. Moreover, notable decreases in the amount of ZIP1 mRNA were observed when individuals were provided with diets containing excess zinc, whereas zinc deficient diets seemed to have increased amounts of ZIP1 mRNA.

Michalczyk and Ackland came up with a hypothetical mechanism model of zinc absorption based on their findings involving the ZIP1 and hZIP4 proteins [59]. To begin with, they proposed that zinc is taken up by differentiated Caco-2 cells via ion channels, such as K^+/Zn^{2+} antiporters, Na^+/Zn^{2+} antiporters, or the hZIP4 transporter. Once inside the cell, the imported zinc is sequestered into vesicles by SLC30/CDF transporters, like ZnT2, ZnT3, and ZnT4. The vesicles containing zinc, commonly known as zincosomes, are then utilized as temporary mineral storage until usage or exocytosis. When cytoplasmic zinc levels decrease, zinc is released from zincosomes via *SLC39A4* transporters. In contrast, high levels of intracellular zinc results in zinc binding with ZIP1 proteins, localized on the zincosomes' membrane, which prevents the release of vesicular zinc into the cytoplasm. The process by which the ZIP1 molecule prevents the release of zinc is unknown. It is important to note that binding events of the ZIP1 are in binding equilibrium and are not an all-or-none event. Zinc binds to or is released by the ZIP1 depending on its intracellular concentration. As a result, less zinc is bound to ZIP1 when cytoplasmic zinc levels decrease, causing the translocation of zinc from the zincosomes to the cytoplasm. In this way, ZIP1 contributes to intracellular zinc homoeostasis [59].

Moreover, Michalczyk and Ackland also proposed the process by which overexpression of the ZIP1 gene affects zinc absorption. The overexpression of ZIP1 in Caco-2 cells would increase the number of ZIP1 molecules that are located on the storage vesicles. Consequently, a greater amount of zinc would be required in order to bind with the additional ZIP1 molecules available to prevent the translocation of zinc from the storage vesicles. Knocking-out the ZIP1 gene would have the opposite effect, where fewer molecules would be available for zinc to bind to; therefore, the saturation of the ZIP1 molecules is reached at a lower intracellular zinc concentration compared to normal conditions [59].

In summary, the ZIP1 protein is not a membrane protein of the apical intestinal membrane and is only found in close proximity of the membrane in mature Caco-2 cells of the intestine. Hence, it indirectly affects zinc absorption in mature Caco-2 cells and functions as a regulatory molecule in order to maintain zinc homoeostasis in the human gut enterocytes.

Furthermore, the presence of zinc binding ligands (ZBLs) in the intestine can provide additional modes of zinc absorption. Zinc can complex with ZBL and be absorbed as part of a ligand molecule. An increase of the amount of ZBL present would result in a greater quantity of zinc-ZBL ligand complexes and an increase in the amount of zinc absorbed. ZBLs may provide a significant additional route for zinc absorption which may be utilized by the body in the absence or limited presence of zinc absorbing proteins, such as hZip4. It is important to note that this is only a theory based on laboratory and clinical research results. This theory still needs to be further tested, while the accurate role of Zinc Binding Ligands in zinc absorption is still to be elucidated.

Following absorption, zinc binds to metallothionein and enters the body's circulation system. After passing through the processing of the liver and kidney, it becomes clear how much zinc remains in the body and how much of it is excreted. It appears that the first stage of zinc absorption is deficient in patients with AE, which is caused by the absence of the hZip4 Zn transporter that is responsible for the absorption of zinc by intestinal cells, as zinc cannot passively diffuse across the apical intestinal membrane. Thus, most of the ingested zinc is excreted after passing through the digestive tract without being absorbed by the individual's body (Fig. 2.4) [14].

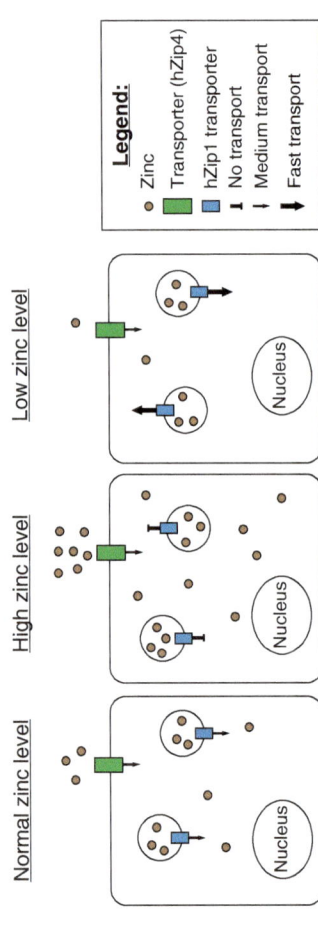

FIGURE 2.4 A model for how the hZIP1 protein operates as an intercellular zinc sensor in intestinal epithelial cells (Caco-2 cells) and maintains intercellular homoeostasis. First, zinc is taken up by membrane transporters, such as hZIP4, and then hZIP1 regulates the release of zinc from the zinc-storage vacuoles, known as zincosomes, in order to maintain a homeostasis intracellular concentration of zinc

References

1. Van Wouwe JP. Clinical and laboratory assessment of zinc deficiency in Dutch children. A review. Biol Trace Elem Res. 1995; 49(2-3):211–25.
2. Küry S, et al. Identification of SLC39A4, a gene involved in acrodermatitis enteropathica. Nat Genet. 2002;31(3):239–40.
3. Schmitt S, et al. An update on mutations of the SLC39A4 gene in acrodermatitis enteropathica. Hum Mutat. 2009;30(6): 926–33.
4. Wang K, et al. A novel member of a zinc transporter family is defective in acrodermatitis enteropathica. Am J Hum Genet. 2002;71(1):66–73.
5. Guilbert JJ. The world health report 2002 – reducing risks, promoting healthy life. Educ Health (Abingdon). 2003;16(2):230.
6. Prasad AS. Discovery of human zinc deficiency: its impact on human health and disease. Adv Nutr. 2013;4(2):176–90.
7. Brown KH, et al. International Zinc Nutrition Consultative Group (IZiNCG) technical document #1. Assessment of the risk of zinc deficiency in populations and options for its control. Food Nutr Bull. 2004;25(1 Suppl 2):S99–203.
8. Prasad AS. Clinical and biochemical spectrum of zinc deficiency in human subjects. 1982.
9. Shrimpton R, et al. Zinc deficiency: what are the most appropriate interventions? BMJ. 2005;330(7487):347–9.
10. Brewer GJ, Prasad AS. Zinc metabolism. Current aspects in health and disease. New York: Alan R. Liss, Inc; 1977.
11. Hambidge KM, Walravens PA. Zinc deficiency in infants and preadolescent children. In: Trace elements in human health and disease, vol. 1. New York: Academic; 1976. p. 21–32.
12. Prasad AS. Clinical manifestations of zinc deficiency. Annu Rev Nutr. 1985;5(1):341–63.
13. Danbolt N, Closs K. Akrodermatitis enteropathica. Acta Derm Venerol. 1942;23:127–69.
14. Neldner KH, Hambidge KM. Zinc therapy of acrodermatitis enteropathica. N Engl J Med. 1975;292(17):879–82.
15. Evans GW, Johnson PE. Characterization and quantitation of a zinc-binding ligand in human milk. Pediatr Res. 1980;14(7): 876–80.
16. Rebello T, Lonnerdal B, Hurley LS. Picolinic acid in milk, pancreatic juice, and intestine: inadequate for role in zinc absorption. Am J Clin Nutr. 1982;35(1):1–5.

17. Bailey MM, et al. Effects of pre- and postnatal exposure to chromium picolinate or picolinic acid on neurological development in CD-1 mice. Biol Trace Elem Res. 2008;124(1):70–82.
18. Seal CJ, Heaton FW. Chemical factors affecting the intestinal absorption of zinc in vitro and in vivo. Br J Nutr. 1983;50(2): 317–24.
19. Eckhert CD, et al. Zinc binding: a difference between human and bovine milk. Science. 1977;195(4280):789–90.
20. Casey CE, Walravens PA, Hambidge KM. Availability of zinc: loading tests with human milk, cow's milk, and infant formulas. Pediatrics. 1981;68(3):394–6.
21. Casey CE, Hambidge KM, Walravens PA. Zinc binding in human duodenal secretions. J Pediatr. 1979;95(6):1008–10.
22. Cousins RJ, Smith KT. Zinc-binding properties of bovine and human milk in vitro: influence of changes in zinc content. Am J Clin Nutr. 1980;33(5):1083–7.
23. Lonnerdal B. Dietary factors influencing zinc absorption. J Nutr. 2000;130(5S Suppl):1378S–83.
24. Sandstrom B. Dose dependence of zinc and manganese absorption in man. Proc Nutr Soc. 1992;51(2):211–8.
25. Sandstrom B, Cederblad A, Lonnerdal B. Zinc absorption from human milk, cow's milk, and infant formulas. Am J Dis Child. 1983;137(8):726–9.
26. Scholmerich J, et al. Bioavailability of zinc from zinc-histidine complexes. II. Studies on patients with liver cirrhosis and the influence of the time of application. Am J Clin Nutr. 1987;45(6): 1487–91.
27. Henkin RI, et al. A syndrome of acute zinc loss. Cerebellar dysfunction, mental changes, anorexia, and taste and smell dysfunction. Arch Neurol. 1975;32(11):745–51.
28. Lonnerdal B, Chen CL. Effects of formula protein level and ratio on infant growth, plasma amino acids and serum trace elements. II. Follow-up formula. Acta Paediatr Scand. 1990;79(3):266–73.
29. Hegenauer J, et al. Iron-supplemented cow milk. Identification and spectral properties of iron bound to casein micelles. J Agric Food Chem. 1979;27(6):1294–301.
30. Hurrell RF, et al. Iron absorption in humans as influenced by bovine milk proteins. Am J Clin Nutr. 1989;49(3):546–52.
31. Hansen M, Sandstrom B, Lonnerdal B. The effect of casein phosphopeptides on zinc and calcium absorption from high phytate infant diets assessed in rat pups and Caco-2 cells. Pediatr Res. 1996;40(4):547–52.

32. Hansen M, et al. Casein phosphopeptides improve zinc and calcium absorption from rice-based but not from whole-grain infant cereal. J Pediatr Gastroenterol Nutr. 1997;24(1):56–62.

33. Menard MP, Cousins RJ. Effect of citrate, glutathione and picolinate on zinc transport by brush border membrane vesicles from rat intestine. J Nutr. 1983;113(8):1653–6.

34. Hurley LS, Lonnerdal B, Stanislowski AG. Zinc citrate, human milk, and acrodermatitis enteropathica. Lancet. 1979;1(8117):677–8.

35. Sang N, et al. Postsynaptically synthesized prostaglandin E2 (PGE2) modulates hippocampal synaptic transmission via a presynaptic PGE2 EP2 receptor. J Neurosci. 2005;25(43):9858–70.

36. Solomons NW, Jacob R. Studies on the bioavailability of zinc in humans: effects of heme and nonheme iron on the absorption of zinc. Am J Clin Nutr. 1981;34(4):475–82.

37. Yip R, et al. Does iron supplementation compromise zinc nutrition in healthy infants? Am J Clin Nutr. 1985;42(4):683–7.

38. Palmiter RD, Findley SD. Cloning and functional characterization of a mammalian zinc transporter that confers resistance to zinc. EMBO J. 1995;14(4):639–49.

39. Palmiter RD, Cole TB, Findley SD. ZnT-2, a mammalian protein that confers resistance to zinc by facilitating vesicular sequestration. EMBO J. 1996;15(8):1784–91.

40. Huang L, Gitschier J. A novel gene involved in zinc transport is deficient in the lethal milk mouse. Nat Genet. 1997;17(3):292–7.

41. Küry S, et al. Expression pattern, genomic structure and evaluation of the human SLC30A4 gene as a candidate for acrodermatitis enteropathica. Hum Genet. 2001;109(2):178–85.

42. Cragg RA, et al. A novel zinc-regulated human zinc transporter, hZTL1, is localized to the enterocyte apical membrane. J Biol Chem. 2002;277(25):22789–97.

43. Wang K, et al. Homozygosity mapping places the acrodermatitis enteropathica gene on chromosomal region 8q24.3. Am J Hum Genet. 2001;68(4):1055–60.

44. Küry S, et al. Mutation spectrum of human SLC39A4 in a panel of patients with acrodermatitis enteropathica. Hum Mutat. 2003;22(4):337–8.

45. Grotz N, et al. Identification of a family of zinc transporter genes from Arabidopsis that respond to zinc deficiency. Proc Natl Acad Sci. 1998;95(12):7220–4.

46. Eng BH, et al. Sequence analyses and phylogenetic characterization of the ZIP family of metal ion transport proteins. J Membr Biol. 1998;166(1):1–7.

47. Guerinot ML, Eide D. Zeroing in on zinc uptake in yeast and plants. Curr Opin Plant Biol. 1999;2(3):244–9.

48. Gaither LA, Eide DJ. The human ZIP1 transporter mediates zinc uptake in human K562 erythroleukemia cells. J Biol Chem. 2001;276(25):22258–64.

49. Kasana S, Din J, Maret W. Genetic causes and gene-nutrient interactions in mammalian zinc deficiencies: acrodermatitis enteropathica and transient neonatal zinc deficiency as examples. J Trace Elem Med Biol. 2014;29C:47–62.

50. Küry S, et al. Clinical utility gene card for: acrodermatitis enteropathica. Eur J Hum Genet. 2012;20(3):1–4.

51. Kim B-E, et al. Zn2+-stimulated endocytosis of the mZIP4 zinc transporter regulates its location at the plasma membrane. J Biol Chem. 2004;279(6):4523–30.

52. Andrews GK. Regulation and function of Zip4, the acrodermatitis enteropathica gene. Biochem Soc Trans. 2008;36(Pt 6): 1242–6.

53. Dufner-Beattie J, et al. The acrodermatitis enteropathica gene ZIP4 encodes a tissue-specific, zinc-regulated zinc transporter in mice. J Biol Chem. 2003;278(35):33474–81.

54. Dufner-Beattie J, et al. The mouse acrodermatitis enteropathica gene Slc39a4 (Zip4) is essential for early development and heterozygosity causes hypersensitivity to zinc deficiency. Hum Mol Genet. 2007;16(12):1391–9.

55. Geiser J, et al. A mouse model of acrodermatitis enteropathica: loss of intestine zinc transporter ZIP4 (Slc39a4) disrupts the stem cell niche and intestine integrity. PLoS Genet. 2012;8(6), e1002766.

56. Kambe T, Andrews GK. Novel proteolytic processing of the ectodomain of the zinc transporter ZIP4 (SLC39A4) during zinc deficiency is inhibited by acrodermatitis enteropathica mutations. Mol Cell Biol. 2009;29(1):129–39.

57. Wang F, et al. Acrodermatitis enteropathica mutations affect transport activity, localization and zinc-responsive trafficking of the mouse ZIP4 zinc transporter. Hum Mol Genet. 2004;13(5):563–71.

58. Küry S, et al. A nine-year experience with the genetic testing of the rare disease acrodermatitis enteropathica; (Abstract #1062T). 2011: Presented at the 12th International Congress of Human Genetics/61st annual meeting of The American Society of Human Genetics, 13 Oct 2011. Montreal.

59. Michalczyk AA, Ackland ML. hZip1 (hSLC39A1) regulates zinc homoeostasis in gut epithelial cells. Genes Nutr. 2013;8(5): 475–86.

60. Küry S, et al. Deciphering the genetics of inherited zinc deficiencies; (Abstract #P01.132). 2013: Presented at the European Human Genetic Conference 2013, 8–11 June 2013. Paris.

61. Chowanadisai W, Lönnerdal B, Kelleher SL. Identification of a mutation in SLC30A2 (ZnT-2) in women with low milk zinc concentration that results in transient neonatal zinc deficiency. J Biol Chem. 2006;281(51):39699–707.

62. Itsumura N, et al. Compound heterozygous mutations in SLC30A2/ZnT2 results in low milk zinc concentrations: a novel mechanism for zinc deficiency in a breast-fed infant. PLoS One. 2013;8(5), e64045.

63. Lasry I, et al. A dominant negative heterozygous G87R mutation in the zinc transporter, ZnT-2 (SLC30A2), results in transient neonatal zinc deficiency. J Biol Chem. 2012;287(35):29348–61.

64. Lova Navarro M, et al. Transient neonatal zinc deficiency due to a new autosomal dominant mutation in gene SLC30A2 (ZnT-2). Pediatr Dermatol. 2014;31(2):251–2.

65. Miletta MC, et al. Transient neonatal zinc deficiency caused by a heterozygous G87R mutation in the zinc transporter ZnT-2 (SLC30A2) gene in the mother highlighting the importance of Zn 2. Int J Endocrinol. 2013;2013.

66. Kelleher SL, et al. Mapping the zinc-transporting system in mammary cells: molecular analysis reveals a phenotype-dependent zinc-transporting network during lactation. J Cell Physiol. 2012;227(4):1761–70.

67. Fukada T, Kambe T. Molecular and genetic features of zinc transporters in physiology and pathogenesis. Metallomics. 2011;3(7):662–74.

68. Kambe T, Weaver BP, Andrews GK. The genetics of essential metal homeostasis during development. Genesis. 2008;46(4):214–28.

69. Lichten LA, Cousins RJ. Mammalian zinc transporters: nutritional and physiologic regulation. Annu Rev Nutr. 2009;29: 153–76.

70. Huang L, Tepaamorndech S. The SLC30 family of zinc transporters–A review of current understanding of their biological and pathophysiological roles. Mol Aspects Med. 2013;34(2):548–60.

71. Palmiter RD, Huang L. Efflux and compartmentalization of zinc by members of the SLC30 family of solute carriers. Pflugers Arch. 2004;447(5):744–51.

72. Liuzzi JP, Cousins RJ. Mammalian zinc transporters. Annu Rev Nutr. 2004;24:151–72.

73. Bloß T, Clemens S, Nies DH. Characterization of the ZAT1p zinc transporter from Arabidopsis thaliana in microbial model organisms and reconstituted proteoliposomes. Planta. 2002;214(5): 783–91.
74. Michalczyk AA, et al. Constitutive expression of hZnT4 zinc transporter in human breast epithelial cells. Biochem J. 2002;364(Pt 1):105–13.
75. Zhao H, Eide D. The yeast ZRT1 gene encodes the zinc transporter protein of a high-affinity uptake system induced by zinc limitation. Proc Natl Acad Sci. 1996;93(6):2454–8.
76. Jiang Y, et al. Genome wide identification, phylogeny and expression of zinc transporter genes in common carp. PLoS One. 2014;9(12), e116043.
77. Martin AB, et al. Gastric and colonic zinc transporter ZIP11 (Slc39a11) in mice responds to dietary zinc and exhibits nuclear localization. J Nutr. 2013;143(12):1882–8.
78. Yu Y, et al. Characterization of the GufA subfamily member SLC39A11/Zip11 as a zinc transporter. J Nutr Biochem. 2013;24(10):1697–708.
79. Liuzzi JP, Blanchard RK, Cousins RJ. Differential regulation of zinc transporter 1, 2, and 4 mRNA expression by dietary zinc in rats. J Nutr. 2001;131(1):46–52.
80. McMahon RJ, Cousins RJ. Regulation of the zinc transporter ZnT-1 by dietary zinc. Proc Natl Acad Sci. 1998;95(9):4841–6.
81. Hambidge KM, et al. Changes in zinc absorption during development. J Pediatr. 2006;149(5 Suppl):S64–8.
82. Zemann N, et al. Differentiation-and polarization-dependent zinc tolerance in Caco-2 cells. Eur J Nutr. 2011;50(5):379–86.
83. Franklin R, et al. Human ZIP1 is a major zinc uptake transporter for the accumulation of zinc in prostate cells. J Inorg Biochem. 2003;96(2):435–42.

Chapter 3
Analysis of Disorder

3.1 Clinical Forms of AE

There are two main forms of AE identified that are clinically distinguishable from each other. The first form of the disorder is an acquired form resulting from a dietary zinc deficiency that resolves upon zinc repletion. The other form is an inheritable disease caused by a mutation in the SLC39A4 gene, which codes for the hZip4 Zn transporter protein, and it is inherited in an autosomal recessive pattern. One or more of its symptoms are often observed in the later stages of the disorder [1].

3.2 Nomenclature of Zinc Deficiencies

AE was identified for the first time by Brandt in 1936 [2]. In 1942, Danbolt and Closs categorized a group of symptoms as AE [3].

Furthermore, it was discovered that AE, which is an autosomal recessive inheritable disorder caused by a mutation in the gene coding for the hZip4 Zn transporter, which is necessary for zinc absorption in the intestine [4]. There have been reports of AE from all around the world and it is not specific to any gender or age [5].

P. Khan Mohammad Beigi, E. Maverakis,
Acrodermatitis Enteropathica: A Clinician's Guide,
DOI 10.1007/978-3-319-17819-6_3,
© Springer International Publishing Switzerland 2015

There are two known types of zinc deficiency disorders which have AE-like symptoms: these disorders can either be hereditary or acquired.

- *Hereditary Acrodermatitis Enteropathica*: this hereditary disorder is autosomal recessive and exclusively affects infants. It diminishes the intestinal uptake of zinc due to the absence of a zinc transporter called hZip4. Skin eruptions (dermatitis), alopecia, and persistent diarrhea are its distinctive symptoms. It can be fatal for infants if it is not diagnosed and treated early and properly [4, 6, 7]. Adult cases are rare and are chronic cases of AE that appear during early infancy of the patient [3].
- *Acquired Non-hereditary Zinc disorders*:
  - Acquired zinc deficiency in newborns is often caused by insufficient zinc levels in maternal breast milk. One example is mutation of *SLC30A2* [8, 9].
  - Pseudo-Acrodermatitis Enteropathica disorder is often not associated with a primary deficiency of zinc. Rather, it is caused by metabolic disorders such as methylmalonic acid productivity disorder, multiple carboxylase disorder, and fatty acid and amino acid deficiencies like Hartnup disease [10–13]. Other conditions such as prolonged total parenteral nutrition, excessive alcohol ingestion, and penicillamine therapy have also been reported to have caused zinc deficiency [14].
  - There have been rare reports of spontaneous improvement of zinc deficiency patients who reach puberty [15], which is likely not true AE but AE-like cases therefore not due to *SLC39A4* mutations.

3.3   Acquired Non-hereditary Zinc Deficiency

As researchers conduct more studies on the biochemical role of zinc in human physiology, they are beginning to discover that zinc deficiency disorders are not simple genetic problems. Because of the researches and studies conducted on hereditary AE, the diagnosis of other diseases and disorders

associated with zinc deficiency have become less compli-
cated. Acquired zinc deficiency has been reported mainly in
two different forms. One form is reported to occur in infants
feeding on zinc deficient maternal milk and the other form is
seen in individuals that are suffering from a metabolic deficiency that has zinc deficiency as a side effect. It is important
to note that any chronic catabolic disorder can cause zinc
deficiency: a few examples are methylmalonic acid productivity disorder, multiple carboxylase disorder, and fatty acid and
amino acid deficiencies. Individuals with alcoholism are particularly prone to zinc deficiency and the clinical condition of
these patients depends on the severity and duration of their
zinc deficiency as well as their age [13]. The mechanism by
which alcohol consumption induces hyperzincuria is not fully
understood, but it may be as a result of alcohol's direct effect
on the renal tubules [16, 17]. Studies show significant increase
in renal clearance of zinc in alcoholics, which resulted in
reduction of the individuals' serum zinc levels. It is important
for clinicians to note that excessive ingestion of alcohol may
cause severe zinc deficiency [18].

One main clinical differentiation between Hereditary AE
and acquired zinc deficiency is that it is possible to stop zinc
supplementation in patients with acquired zinc deficiency
without the disease recurring. In contrast, in AE, the zinc
supplementation is usually given for life because of the defective zinc absorption in the small intestine [19, 20].

3.3.1   Zinc Deficient Maternal Breast Milk

Acquired zinc deficiency in newborns is often caused by
insufficient zinc levels in the maternal breast milk resulting in
hypozincemia in the newborns. Because of their rapid rate of
growth, normal infants require large amounts of zinc compared to adults. This is accentuated in premature infants who
require even more zinc [20]. As a result, premature infants
are more susceptible to acquired zinc deficiency. These transient forms of zinc deficiency may be due for instance to
mutations in SLC30A2 [21].

Maternal milk is normally a good source of zinc; however, in these cases the maternal milk has a low zinc concentration that cannot be corrected by oral zinc supplementation. This is because the zinc-secreting mechanism of the mammary glands is defective. For instance in a literature case, a nursing mother, whose milk zinc level was low at 6 μmol/L while her serum zinc level was normal at 15 μmol/L, was subjected to 220 mg of zinc sulfate three times a day for a week and no change was observed in her milk zinc level [20]. This case is evident of a defective zinc-secreting mechanism since the maternal breast milk zinc concentration should be higher than those of the maternal serum for the purpose of meeting the infant's growth and developmental requirements [8]. Moreover, this zinc deficiency condition can be clinically distinguished from AE since its symptoms only develop during breast feeding and do not recur after weaning [22].

Recent genetic studies have indicated that mutations in the *SLC30A2* gene, which codes for the ZnT2 transporter protein, could be the cause for this defective zinc secretion. When functional, the transporter, located in mammary epithelial cells, is responsible for secretion of zinc into breast milk during lactation [23, 24]. Figure 3.1 illustrates the predicted molecular structure of the hZnT2 protein. As illustrated by the figure the transporter is predicted to have 6 transmembrane domains with a long histidine loop between transmembrane domains IV and V, which is likely to be a zinc-binding region [8, 25, 26].

When defective, it results in low zinc secretion into breast milk causing the infant who feeds on the milk to develop zinc deficiency. Interestingly, it was found that lactating mothers that were homozygous for the *SLC30A2* mutation or heterozygous carriers of the *SLC30A2* mutations also had low milk zinc levels, which is suggestive of haploinsufficiency [8]. In mouse, homozygous mutations of *SLC30A4* in lactating mothers cause zinc deficiency in their pups resulting in the *lethal milk* phenotype [27], which was previously discussed in the etiology section. These infants were successfully treated

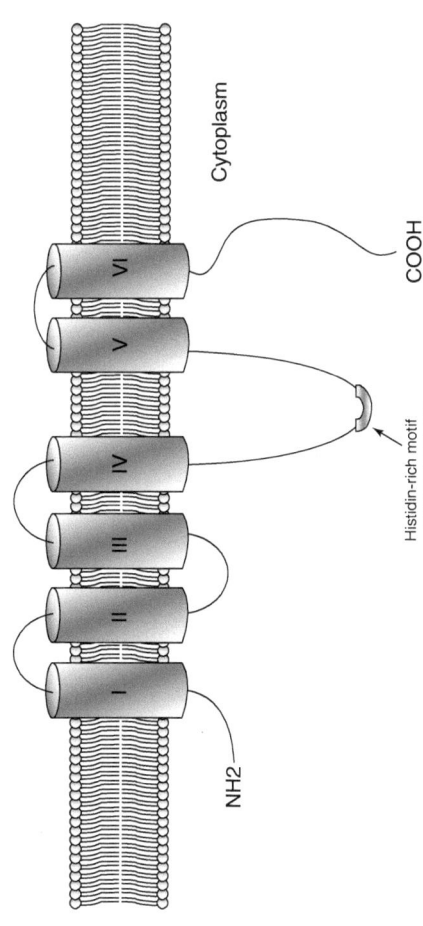

FIGURE 3.1 Predicted structure of ZnT2 protein. The dark grey barrels represent the transmembrane domains. It is characterized by 6 transmembrane domains organized into two blocks of 4 and 2 separated by a histidine-rich cytoplasmic metal-binding site

with the addition of zinc to their diets. It is important to note that as these infants grew up and discontinued breast milk, they no longer needed supplemental zinc since they were not actually suffering from a hereditary zinc disorder and their symptoms were attributed to purely dietary deficiency during infancy.

3.3.2   Zinc Deficiency Caused by Metabolism Disorders

Acquired zinc deficiency caused by metabolism disorders can occur in any age and it is usually not associated with a primary deficiency of zinc. As a result, *SLC39A4* mutations do not play a role in this type of zinc deficiency. The different metabolic disorders that result in zinc deficiency were mentioned in section 3.2 and will be discussed in detail in the differential diagnosis section in Chap. 5.

Moreover, the signs and symptoms of acquired zinc deficiency have been reported as skin lesions such as eczematoid plaques, hyperkeratotic plaques, alopecia, nail dystrophy, glossitis, stomatitis [28] as well as neurological changes such as insomnia, anorexia, lethargy, low spirits, and lack of self-interest [29–31]. Low serum zinc levels and high urine zinc concentration are other indicators of acquired zinc deficiency [29]. For treatment, patients were prescribed zinc supplementation which resulted in the clearing of their symptoms and treatment of their acquired zinc deficiency [28, 29]. It is interesting to note that hereditary AE also shares some of the symptoms of acquired zinc deficiency. As a result, acrodermatitis enteropathica should not be diagnosed unless other possible factors that may lead to zinc deficiency have been excluded.

Clinicians should be mindful of the fact that any patient who is receiving long-term total parenteral nutrition (TPN) without supplementation of trace elements is likely to become deficient in them [28, 32].

References

1. Danbolt N. Acrodermatitis enteropathica. Br J Dermatol. 1979;100(1):37–40.
2. Brandt T. Dermatitis in children with disturbances of the general condition and the absorption of food elements. Acta Derm. 1936;17:513–46.
3. Danbolt N, Closs K. Akrodermatitis enteropathica. Acta Derm Venerol. 1942;23:127–69.
4. Michalczyk AA, Ackland ML. hZip1 (hSLC39A1) regulates zinc homoeostasis in gut epithelial cells. Genes Nutr. 2013;8(5):475–86.
5. Van Wouwe JP. Clinical and laboratory assessment of zinc deficiency in Dutch children. A review. Biol Trace Elem Res. 1995;49(2-3):211–25.
6. Van Wouwe JP. Clinical and laboratory diagnosis of acrodermatitis enteropathica. Eur J Pediatr. 1989;149(1):2–8.
7. Aggett PJ. Acrodermatitis enteropathica. J Inherit Metab Dis. 1983;6 Suppl 1:39–43.
8. Itsumura N, et al. Compound heterozygous mutations in SLC30A2/ZnT2 results in low milk zinc concentrations: a novel mechanism for zinc deficiency in a breast-fed infant. PLoS One. 2013;8(5), e64045.
9. Wessells KR, King JC, Brown KH. Development of a plasma zinc concentration cutoff to identify individuals with severe zinc deficiency based on results from adults undergoing experimental severe dietary zinc restriction and individuals with acrodermatitis enteropathica. J Nutr. 2014;144(8):1204–10.
10. Williams ML, Packman S, Cowan MJ. Alopecia and periorificial dermatitis in biotin-responsive multiple carboxylase deficiency. J Am Acad Dermatol. 1983;9(1):97–103.
11. Norton JA, et al. Amino acid deficiency and the skin rash associated with glucagonoma. Ann Intern Med. 1979;91(2):213–5.
12. Seyhan ME, et al. Acrodermatitis enteropathica-like eruptions in a child with Hartnup disease. Pediatr Dermatol. 2006;23(3):262–5.
13. Montinari M, Parodi A, Rongioletti F. Chapter 13: Aquired nutritional deficiencies. In: Smoller BR, Rongioletti F, editors. Clinical and pathological aspects of skin diseases in endocrine, metabolic, nutritional and deposition disease. New York: Springer; 2010.

14. Prasad AS. Clinical manifestations of zinc deficiency. Annu Rev Nutr. 1985;5(1):341–63.
15. Bronson DM, Barsky R, Barsky S. Acrodermatitis enteropathica. J Am Acad Dermatol. 1983;9(1):140–4.
16. Allan J, Fell G, Russell R. Urinary zinc in hepatic cirrhosis. Scott Med J. 1975;20(3):109–11.
17. Gudbjarnason S, Prasad AS. Cardiac metabolism in experimental alcoholism. Biochem Clin Aspect Alcohol Metab.1969;101:266.
18. WEISMANN K, et al. Chronic zinc deficiency syndrome in a beer drinker with a Billroth II resection. Int J Dermatol. 1976;15(10):757–61.
19. Evans G, Johnson P. Zinc-binding factor in acrodermatitis enteropathica. Lancet. 1976;308(7998):1310.
20. Connors TJ, Czarnecki D, Haskett MI. Acquired zinc deficiency in a breast-fed premature infant. Arch Dermatol. 1983;119(4): 319–21.
21. Zattra E, Belloni Fortina A. Transient symptomatic zinc deficiency resembling acrodermatitis enteropathica in a breast-fed premature infant: case report and brief review of the literature. G Ital Dermatol Venereol. 2013;148(6):699–702.
22. Ackland ML, Michalczyk A. Zinc deficiency and its inherited disorders-a review. Genes Nutr. 2006;1(1):41–9.
23. Chowanadisai W, Lönnerdal B, Kelleher SL. Identification of a mutation in SLC30A2 (ZnT-2) in women with low milk zinc concentration that results in transient neonatal zinc deficiency. J Biol Chem. 2006;281(51):39699–707.
24. Lasry I, et al. A dominant negative heterozygous G87R mutation in the zinc transporter, ZnT-2 (SLC30A2), results in transient neonatal zinc deficiency. J Biol Chem. 2012;287(35):29348–61.
25. Bloß T, Clemens S, Nies DH. Characterization of the ZAT1p zinc transporter from Arabidopsis thaliana in microbial model organisms and reconstituted proteoliposomes. Planta. 2002;214(5):783–91.
26. Maverakis E, et al. Acrodermatitis enteropathica and an overview of zinc metabolism. J Am Acad Dermatol. 2007;56(1): 116–24.
27. Huang L, Gitschier J. A novel gene involved in zinc transport is deficient in the lethal milk mouse. Nat Genet. 1997;17(3):292–7.
28. Tucker SB, et al. Acquired zinc deficiency: cutaneous manifestations typical of acrodermatitis enteropathica. JAMA. 1976; 235(22):2399–402.

29. Ecker RI, Schroeter AL. Acrodermatitis and acquired zinc deficiency. Arch Dermatol. 1978;114(6):937–9.
30. Moynahan E. Zinc deficiency and disturbances of mood and visual behaviour. Lancet. 1976;307(7950):91.
31. Kay R, Tasman-Jones C. Zinc deficiency and intravenous feeding. Lancet. 1975;306(7935):605–6.
32. Vloten W, Bos L. Skin lesions in acquired zinc deficiency due to parenteral nutrition. Dermatology. 1978;156(3):175–83.

Chapter 4
Clinical Symptoms

Acrodermatitis Enteropathica symptoms usually begin to appear either within the first few days of life in formula fed infants or immediately upon discontinuation of breastfeeding [1]. Appearance of symptoms after change from breast milk to bovine milk indicates that human milk has a protective role which may be due to presence of low molecular binding agents that increase zinc bioavailability [2]. Common early symptoms of AE include the appearance of perleche (angular chelitis), skin lesions, erythematous patches, plaques of dry and scaly skin, and eczematous plaques on the face, scalp, and genital area: these skin dermatitises deteriorate quickly [1]. The lesions gradually begin emerging inside the mouth and then on the hands and feet, accompanied by paronychia and inflammatory dermatitis on the palms, wrinkles on fingers, as well as scaly skin on the neck [3]. Next, diarrhea is one of the most variable symptoms of AE. If it appears and is exacerbated, it could lead to dehydration and loss of essential minerals and electrolytes; which could result in complications with the clinical treatment [1].

Furthermore, lack of growth is often observed in patients, especially in children approaching puberty, within a few weeks after the appearance of the early symptoms. In addition, hypogonadism is seen to start in male patients. Mental and emotional disorders are also common signs and symptoms of AE although they are nonspecific findings.

P. Khan Mohammad Beigi, E. Maverakis,   39
Acrodermatitis Enteropathica: A Clinician's Guide,
DOI 10.1007/978-3-319-17819-6_4,
© Springer International Publishing Switzerland 2015

Photophobia usually develops gradually and most medical researchers believe that it is associated with retinal protein disorder, which is caused by zinc deficiency. Other symptoms of AE include anorexia, hypogeusia, hyposmia, and anemia [1].

AE is often fatal in infants. The infants that survive either have a mild form of AE or obtain a great amount of zinc through their diet, leading to the infants having less severe symptoms. However, AE usually results in lack of growth, dwarfism, delayed puberty, hypogonadism in males at puberty, skin dermatitis, frequent infections, prolonged wound healing, and mental disorders [4–6].

Classical AE often develops during the first week or month after birth especially when the infant discontinued breast milk. This disorder is characterized by dermatological, gastrointestinal and psychological disorders. With regards to dermatological disorders, skin eruptions and manifestations are often clear symptoms of AE: erythematous, dry, and rough pseudo psoriasis lesions are a few examples of these skin eruptions [1]. These skin manifestations are often found near the mouth, nose, eyes, ears, and perineum and termed periorificial. Pustular and vesicular lesions are the dominant forms of the dermatological symptoms of AE. Perleche is also common and can be an early sign of the disorder. Furthermore, diarrhea, abdominal pain, and foul-smelling stools are usually the first gastrointestinal symptoms of AE. Psychological symptoms include mental depression, excitability, and decreased appetite. In addition, alopecia and visual disorders such as blepharitis, photophobia, and reduced vision have also been reported as secondary symptoms of Acrodermatitis Enteropathica [1]. Treatment with the administration of zinc supplements and diiodohydroxyquin, which has a chemical structure similar to picolinic acid have been effective. Early diagnosis and prescription of zinc supplements are fundamental and necessary to reduce the very high death rate of AE [7] (Fig. 4.1).

FIGURE 4.1 chemical structure of diiodohydroxyquin

References

1. Van Wouwe JP. Clinical and laboratory diagnosis of acrodermatitis enteropathica. Eur J Pediatr. 1989;149(1):2–8.
2. Arnaud J, Favier A. Determination of ultrafilterable zinc in human milk by electrothermal atomic absorption spectrometry. Analyst. 1992;117(10):1593–8.
3. Maverakis E, et al. Acrodermatitis enteropathica and an overview of zinc metabolism. J Am Acad Dermatol. 2007;56(1):116–24.
4. Gehrig KA, Dinulos JG. Acrodermatitis due to nutritional deficiency. Curr Opin Pediatr. 2010;22(1):107–12.
5. Seyhan ME, et al. Acrodermatitis enteropathica-like eruptions in a child with Hartnup disease. Pediatr Dermatol. 2006;23(3):262–5.
6. Sehgal VN, Jain S. Acrodermatitis enteropathica. Clin Dermatol. 2000;18(6):745–8.
7. Puri N. A study of efficacy of oral zinc therapy for acrodermatitis enteropathica. Nasza Dermatolologia Online. 2013;4:162–6.

Chapter 5
Diagnosis

5.1 Laboratory Diagnosis of Zinc Deficiency

Presently, measurement of zinc levels in blood plasma or serum is the simplest and most common way of determining the body's zinc status. However, infections, injuries, and other stress stimuli can alter blood zinc levels and confound the clinical picture when attempting to diagnose AE based on plasma zinc levels. The mechanism for the decreased serum zinc levels observed in the setting of inflammation has not been completely elucidated, but a recent discovery that inter-luekin-6 (IL-6) upregulates the expression of the ZIP14 zinc transporter in murine liver and may contribute to the hypozincemia seen in inflammatory states [1]. In addition, zinc is distributed to different parts of the body; as a result blood zinc levels may not be reflective of the total body stores. Normal levels of zinc in blood plasma range between 70 and 110 μg/dL, while zinc levels in blood serum range from 80 to 120 μg/dL. Under normal conditions, zinc excretion through urine varies but urinary zinc excretion is significantly reduced in individuals with zinc deficiency [2]. Hair zinc levels are also decreased in patients with AE and it was proposed to detect heterozygous carriers of SLC39A4 mutations [3].

There are several steps the clinician can take in order to maximize the accuracy of the serum zinc concentrations when assessing for potential zinc deficiency. Labs should be drawn in

P. Khan Mohammad Beigi, E. Maverakis,
Acrodermatitis Enteropathica: A Clinician's Guide,
DOI 10.1007/978-3-319-17819-6_5,
© Springer International Publishing Switzerland 2015

a fasting patient who has not taken any zinc supplements the day of the laboratory test. The sample should be collected in a trace element-free collection tube, and care should be taken to avoid hemolyzing the sample which may falsely elevate the serum zinc level [4]. Fasting zinc levels should be greater than 70 μg/dL, and will be lowered after meals. Serum zinc levels less than 50 μg/dL are suggestive of potential AE, but true diagnosis requires a supportive clinical picture [5].

In vitro or in vivo zinc absorption tests are performed using zinc radioisotopes: zinc-65 or zinc-69 may be performed as confirmatory measures [6]. It should be emphasized that laboratory techniques are very important in determining accurate test results, since contamination of containers and samples and flawed laboratory techniques can alter the patient's lab results and cause a false diagnosis.

Hyperleukocytosis, anemia, hypertension, as well as low calcium levels, phosphate levels, gastric lipase levels and protease levels are seen in laboratory results of AE patients. In the stool test of these patients, fatty acid content is high (50 % of the cases) and sometimes candida albicans, trichocephalus, and lamblia are found [7].

For patients with borderline laboratory results, a therapeutic trial is recommended to determine if the abnormality is due to a zinc deficiency. This therapeutic trial, also known as a zinc tolerance test, presents an accurate representation of body zinc nutriture and is carried out in the following manner [8, 9]:

1. After a fast, a baseline plasma level is drawn.
2. 220 mg zinc sulfate (50 mg elemental zinc) is orally administered.
3. After 2 h, plasma level is redrawn
4. If plasma zinc is increased by two or three times, then the result is indicative of zinc inadequacy

Furthermore, other tests such as neutrophil alkaline phosphatase activity [10], the enzyme 5'-nucleotidase [11], and erythrocyte metallothionein [12] have been found to present accurate measurements.

5.2   Histopathology

Confounding the diagnostic process, cutaneous lesions of AE do not have specific histopathology. The early skin lesions of AE are characterized by replacement of the granular layer by clear cells and parakeratosis. These skin lesions may have the appearance of eczema or psoriasis. As the condition progresses, the pallor of the upper part of the epidermis becomes more prominent and the parakeratosis is observed to become more confluent. Later on, the pallor is seen to disappear while the psoriasiform appearance still persists [13].

Notable characteristics of AE include the spreading of parakeratosis and psoriatic epidermal hyperkeratosis with large pale keratinocytes on top of lumbar spine and dyscrasia cells, flattened layer of malpighian cells, and absence of granular layer. In addition to its academic advantages, examination of these manifestations and lesions under the electron microscope can be helpful. Furthermore, biopsy examinations can also be conducted in order detect non-specialized changes in enterocytes.

5.3   Biological Diagnosis of Acrodermatitis Enteropathica

Measurement of plasma zinc levels is the most reliable method of determining the amount of zinc present in the patient's body providing that the sample is not hemolyzed or contaminated. However, there have been cases of falsely low levels of zinc caused by acute stress, infections, and myocardial infarction due to zinc redistribution from blood plasma to body tissues making the assessment of zinc status in the body difficult and inaccurate [14]. On average, zinc concentration in serum is 16 % more than that of plasma due to zinc release in the process of blood clotting and from hemolyzed erythrocytes.

In general, plasma zinc levels do not depend on age or sex of the individuals. One exception is zinc levels in infants younger than 6 months that are approximately 25 % less than the normal levels seen in children and adults. Moreover, zinc levels also depend on albumin levels in plasma. As a result, elderly individuals in whom hypoalbuminemia is more common, have lower zinc levels [15]. Furthermore, leukocytes have high zinc content (56.8–168 µg $Zn/10^{10}$ WBC), which is roughly 10 times the amount present in erythrocytes (9.3–15.5 µg $Zn/10^{10}$ RBC). Nevertheless, zinc levels in erythrocytes and hair strands are often used to evaluate zinc status of the body; however, since these cells and tissues have a slow restoration process, measurement of their zinc levels does not properly resemble the body's recent zinc status. The zinc level in neutrophils is a more precise and accurate resemblance of the body's recent zinc status.

Among zinc-dependent metalloproteinase enzymes, qualitative assessment of the activity of alkaline phosphatase present in serum and neutrophils may be useful for evaluating zinc status in the body. In the absence of evidence of liver or bone disease, decrease in alkaline phosphatase activity may indicate zinc deficiency [16]. In 1985, this observation was further supported by the clinical research carried out by Weismann and Hoyer, in which the assessment of the activity of alkaline phosphatase was utilized to diagnose mild cases of zinc deficiency as well as cases of AE [17].

In patients diagnosed with AE, zinc levels in plasma, urine, hair, erythrocytes, and leukocytes, as well as the activity of alkaline phosphatase, ribonuclease, and serum LDH have been observed to decrease. Additionally, a strong correlation was seen between the level of plasma zinc and the activity of alkaline phosphatase. Conversely, the activity of erythrocyte carbonic anhydrase did not show any correlation with plasma zinc levels [16, 18].

In cases of zinc deficiency, plasma zinc levels decrease several weeks before clinical manifestations appear. Generally, when plasma zinc levels reach 60–70 µg/dL, the skin manifestations of the disease begin to appear as roughness and dryness. In most AE patients, zinc levels often reached 10–50 μg/dL before any clinical symptoms began to appear. As previously mentioned, urinary excretion of zinc diminishes in patients that have zinc deficiency disorder; therefore zinc excreted through urine, collected within the first 24 h of patient's admission to hospital or medical clinic, can be useful in the diagnosis provided that the most common causes of second degree hypozincemia such as cirrhosis, sickle cell disease, and uremia are taken into account [19].

5.4 Clinical Diagnosis

Arriving at the diagnosis of AE relies on the ability of the clinician to recognize the constellation of distinct symptoms. However, the presenting signs other than skin lesions often vary with the age of the patient. Clinical findings such as psoriasis manifestations, symmetrical lesions, alopecia, anorexia, neurological disorders, diarrhea, and mood changes have been often reported in infants; while mental retardation, alopecia, weight loss, secondary infections, and growth problems have been reported in toddlers and school aged children.

Laboratory examinations are interpreted in support of the clinical symptoms, but cannot be a substitute in the absence of the appropriate clinical findings. Estimations of zinc levels in serum, urine, and hair are used to diagnose zinc deficiency in individuals. Nevertheless, interpretation of laboratory results is prone to some difficulty because of the potential overlap of the clinical symptoms of AE with coincident findings that may be observed in healthy individuals such as dermatitis. Additionally, low zinc levels in serum, urine, and hair are also observed in other disease and disorders. As a result, the age of the patient and albumin levels of serum are also considered for a more precise and accurate diagnosis. A more specific and accurate laboratory test is often necessary. In vitro or in vivo zinc absorption tests are performed using zinc radioisotopes zinc-65 or zinc-69.

In the absence of diagnostic hypozincemia the above laboratory tests, 3–30 μ mole of zinc per kilogram is prescribed for

5 days. This treatment is especially recommended for infants or children with one or more symptoms of AE. A positive response to this treatment would be a retrospective support of the clinical diagnosis [6, 20].

5.5   Molecular Diagnosis

Confirmation of the diagnosis of AE can be brought by a genetic testing for AE. True AE cases necessarily present either a homozygous or two compound heterozygous mutations of the *SLC39A4* gene [21]. Patients who do not have such mutations are to be considered as presenting AE-like disorders, which can either be acquired or due to a genetic predisposition by a mutation in another gene of zinc homeostasis (zinc transporters or metallothioneins). Certain forms of transient zinc deficiencies may be due to mutations of the SLC30A2 gene [22–26].

5.6   Differential Diagnosis

AE-like symptoms of zinc deficiency, which can have numerous different causes, have been observed in infants who were diagnosed with acquired zinc deficiency [2]. This is because some zinc deficiency disorders like dermatosis are clinically indistinguishable from acrodermatitis enteropathica as a consequence of their overlapping symptoms. For instance, perioral and acral dermatitis are the shared symptoms of dermatosis and AE; and both are seen to markedly improve with the intake of oral zinc supplements [27]. Interestingly, there have been reported cases of patients with AE-like eruptions who were suffering from essential free fatty acid and protein deficiencies as well as mild zinc deficiency. In one particular case, the condition of the patient was improved by total parenteral nutrition including amino acids, albumin, lipid, and zinc. Hence it was inferred that all three elements in concert caused her dermatoses [28, 29]. Zinc and essential fatty acids (EFA) interact in a various ways inside the human body; this may be why their deficiencies have similar symptoms. It has been observed that essential fatty acids are important in zinc absorption. Zinc was found to be necessary for at least two stages in EFA metabolism: the conversion of linoleic acid to gamma-linolenic acid and the mobilisation of dihomo-gamma-linolenic acid (DGLA) for the synthesis of prostaglandins. Zinc may also be important in the conversion of DGLA to arachidonic acid and in arachidonic acid mobilisation [29].

Furthermore, insufficient zinc levels in maternal breast milk were seen to cause skin eruptions, such as erythematous, erosive, and crusted patches and plaques in perioral, scalp, genital, perianal regions of the nursing infants [30, 31]. This insufficiency of zinc in breast milk is usually caused by a disorder affecting uptake of zinc by the mammary gland from maternal serum [31]. Moreover, total parenteral nutrition (TPN) that are zinc free can also lead to skin lesions along with digestive disorders, which can have the appearance of AE symptoms like alopecia, weight loss, and neuropsychiatric and dermatologic symptoms [32, 33].

In addition, other skin eruptions that are not associated with serum zinc level may mimic the symptoms of AE, such as methylmalonic acid productivity disorder, multiple carboxylase disorder, and amino acid deficiency [34, 35]. AE symptoms are also seen in patients suffering from Crohn's disease, enterocolitis, Hartnup disease, cystic fibrosis, as well as in patients undergoing dialysis [20, 36–38].

AE is typically characterized by significant decrease in serum zinc level. It is important to note that the clinical diagnosis of AE may be challenging due to the roughly 15 % overlap in the symptoms of the disorder with healthy individuals and other similar diseases and disorders [2, 39]. For instance in diseases like cystic fibrosis, decreased levels of zinc in serum, urine, and hair may be observed [36]. Additionally, AE-like symptoms such as pellagra eruptions, vomiting, and diarrhea were observed in a patient who was diagnosed with Hartnup disease with a normal isoleucine level [39]. Therefore, multiple and laboratory medical examinations are often conducted for a more accurate diagnosis. One example is the in-vivo or in-vitro zinc uptake test which is carried out with radioisotopes zinc-65 and zinc-69 [40, 41]. Recently, genetic testing has been used in order to distinguish between true AE and AE-like disorders [42]. This matter will be examined in detail in the upcoming sections.

Recently, there have been reports of preterm infants suffering from dermatitis, suspected of having AE; however, it was determined that these infants' symptoms were associated with insufficient biotin metabolism or biotinidase deficiency [43].

The symptoms of Acrodermatitis Enteropathica in children can often be confused with malnutrition or kwashiorkor. If Acrodermatitis Enteropathica is not treated and has a continuous and progressive process, it can cause long-term weakness, frequent infections, and even fatality within 4–5 years. However, improvements are sometimes observed which are mainly due to improved nutrition.

Furthermore, differential diagnosis with the following disease and disorders should also be mentioned:

- Epidermolysis bullosa
- Eczema
- Pyoderma gangrenosum
- seborrheic dermatitis
- Dermatitis Herpetiformis (Duhring's disease)
- Stevens-Johnson syndrome
- Erythema multiforme
- Reiter's syndrome
- Finger manifestations of Acrodermatitis Hallopeau
- Psoriasis Vulgaris
- Apthous ulcers
- Partial biotinidase zinc deficiency
- Atropic dermatitis

References

1. Liuzzi JP, et al. Interleukin-6 regulates the zinc transporter Zip14 in liver and contributes to the hypozincemia of the acute-phase response. Proc Natl Acad Sci U S A. 2005;102(19):6843–8.
2. Van Wouwe JP. Clinical and laboratory diagnosis of acrodermatitis enteropathica. Eur J Pediatr. 1989;149(1):2–8.
3. Jamall IS, Ally KM, Yusuf S. Acrodermatitis enteropathica. Biol Trace Elem Res. 2006;114(1-3):93–105.
4. Maverakis E, et al. Acrodermatitis enteropathica and an overview of zinc metabolism. J Am Acad Dermatol. 2007;56(1): 116–24.
5. King JC, et al. Daily variation in plasma zinc concentrations in women fed meals at six-hour intervals. J Nutr. 1994;124(4):508–16.
6. Aggett PJ. Acrodermatitis enteropathica. J Inherit Metab Dis. 1983;6 Suppl 1:39–43.
7. Ishibashi Y, et al. Abnormalities of fecal flora in patients with acrodermatitis enteropathica. J Dermatol. 1985;12(3):219–25.
8. Werbach MR. Nutritional influences on illness. Tarzana: Third Line Press; 1993.
9. Capel ID, et al. The assessment of zinc status by the zinc tolerance test in various groups of patients. Clin Biochem. 1982;15(5): 257–60.
10. Prasad A. Laboratory diagnosis of zinc deficiency. J Am Coll Nutr. 1985;4(6):591–8.
11. Bales CW, et al. Marginal zinc deficiency in older adults: responsiveness of zinc status indicators. J Am Coll Nutr. 1994;13(5):455–62.
12. Lee D-Y, COUSINS RJ. Erythrocyte metallothionein response to dietary zinc in humans. 1993.
13. Brandt T. Dermatitis in children with disturbances of the general condition and the absorption of food elements. Acta Derm. 1936;17:513–46.
14. Katayama T, et al. Serum zinc concentration in acute myocardial infarction. Angiology. 1990;41(6):479–85.
15. Obara H, Tomite Y, Doi M. Serum trace elements in tube-fed neurological dysphagia patients correlate with nutritional indices but do not correlate with trace element intakes: case of patients receiving enough trace elements intake. Clin Nutr. 2008;27(4):587–93.

16. Van Wouwe JP. Clinical and laboratory assessment of zinc deficiency in Dutch children. A review. Biol Trace Elem Res. 1995; 49(2-3):211–25.
17. Weismann K, Høyer H. Serum alkaline phosphatase activity in acrodermatitis enteropathica: an index of the serum zinc level. Acta Derm Venereol. 1978;59(1):89–90.
18. Evans GW, Johnson PE. Characterization and quantitation of a zinc-binding ligand in human milk. Pediatr Res. 1980;14(7): 876–80.
19. Wessells KR, King JC, Brown KH. Development of a plasma zinc concentration cutoff to identify individuals with severe zinc deficiency based on results from adults undergoing experimental severe dietary zinc restriction and individuals with acrodermatitis enteropathica. J Nutr. 2014;144(8):1204–10.
20. Seyhan ME, et al. Acrodermatitis enteropathica-like eruptions in a child with Hartnup disease. Pediatr Dermatol. 2006;23(3):262–5.
21. Küry S, et al. Clinical utility gene card for: acrodermatitis enteropathica. Eur J Hum Genet. 2012;20(3):1–4.
22. Chowanadisai W, Lönnerdal B, Kelleher SL. Identification of a mutation in SLC30A2 (ZnT-2) in women with low milk zinc concentration that results in transient neonatal zinc deficiency. J Biol Chem. 2006;281(51):39699–707.
23. Itsumura N, et al. Compound heterozygous mutations in SLC30A2/ZnT2 results in low milk zinc concentrations: a novel mechanism for zinc deficiency in a breast-fed infant. PLoS One. 2013;8(5), e64045.
24. Lasry I, et al. A dominant negative heterozygous G87R mutation in the zinc transporter, ZnT-2 (SLC30A2), results in transient neonatal zinc deficiency. J Biol Chem. 2012;287(35):29348–61.
25. Lova Navarro M, et al. Transient neonatal zinc deficiency due to a New autosomal dominant mutation in gene SLC30A2 (ZnT-2). Pediatr Dermatol. 2014;31(2):251–2.
26. Miletta MC, et al. Transient neonatal zinc deficiency caused by a heterozygous G87R mutation in the zinc transporter ZnT-2 (SLC30A2) gene in the mother highlighting the importance of Zn 2. Int J Endocrinol. 2013;2013.
27. Shim JH, JK, Park HY, Lee DY, Yang JM. P212: Acrodermatitis enteropathica-like dermatosis secondary to acquired zinc deficiency. Unknown Journal. 2014;66:372.
28. Kim YJ, et al. Acrodermatitis enteropathica-like eruption associated with combined nutritional deficiency. J Korean Med Sci. 2005;20(5):908–11.

29. Horrobin DF, Cunnane SC. Interactions between zinc, essential fatty acids and prostaglandins: relevance to acrodermatitis enteropathica, total parenteral nutrition, the glucagonoma syndrome, diabetes, anorexia nervosa and sickle cell anaemia. Med Hypotheses. 1980;6(3):277–96.

30. Glover MT, Atherton DJ. Transient zinc deficiency in two full-term breast-fed siblings associated with low maternal breast milk zinc concentration. Pediatr Dermatol. 1988;5(1):10–3.

31. Laureano A, et al. Transient symptomatic zinc deficiency in a pre-term exclusively breast-fed infant. Dermatol Online J. 2014;20(2): 14–7.

32. Prasad AS. Discovery of human zinc deficiency: its impact on human health and disease. Adv Nutr. 2013;4(2):176–90.

33. Guidelines for essential trace element preparations for parenteral use. A statement by an expert panel. AMA Department of Foods and Nutrition. JAMA. 1979;241(19):2051–4.

34. Williams ML, Packman S, Cowan MJ. Alopecia and periorificial dermatitis in biotin-responsive multiple carboxylase deficiency. J Am Acad Dermatol. 1983;9(1):97–103.

35. Norton JA, et al. Amino acid deficiency and the skin rash associated with glucagonoma. Ann Intern Med. 1979;91(2):213–5.

36. Hansen RC, Lemen R, Revsin B. Cystic fibrosis manifesting with acrodermatitis enteropathica-like eruption. Association with essential fatty acid and zinc deficiencies. Arch Dermatol. 1983;119(1):51–5.

37. Dalgic B, Egritas O. Gray hair and acrodermatitis enteropathica-like dermatitis: an unexpected presentation of cystic fibrosis. Eur J Pediatr. 2011;170(10):1305–8.

38. Gehrig KA, Dinulos JG. Acrodermatitis due to nutritional deficiency. Curr Opin Pediatr. 2010;22(1):107–12.

39. Sehgal VN, Jain S. Acrodermatitis enteropathica. Clin Dermatol. 2000;18(6):745–8.

40. Danbolt N. Acrodermatitis enteropathica. Br J Dermatol. 1979;100(1):37–40.

41. Montinari M, Parodi A, Rongioletti F. Chapter 13: Aquired nutritional deficiencies. In: Smoller BR, Rongioletti F, editors. Clinical and pathological aspects of skin diseases in endocrine, metabolic, nutritional and deposition disease. New York: Springer; 2010.

42. Küry S, et al. Identification of SLC39A4, a gene involved in acrodermatitis enteropathica. Nat Genet. 2002;31(3):239–40.

43. Wolf B, et al. Biotinidase deficiency: the enzymatic defect in late-onset multiple carboxylase deficiency. Clin Chim Acta. 1983; 131(3):273–81.

Chapter 6
Disease Course
and Treatment

The natural history of AE is that of a slowly progressive disease, often presenting in mild form. Untreated, AE is potentially fatal and one third of these reported cases have led to patient death.

6.1   Treatment

To begin with, successful treatment of Acrodermatitis Enteropathica with the oral administration of diodoquin (diiodohydroxyquinoline) was first reported by Dillaha et al. in 1953 [1]. Later on, clioquinol, which is also known as iodochlorhydroxyquin or 5-chloro-7-iodo-quinolin-8-ol, was generally prescribed as the main treatment for AE. There were reports that this drug enhances zinc absorption in patients. However, the use of clioquinol was epidemiologically linked to subacute myelo-optic neuropathy (SMON), which is characterized by peripheral neuropathy and blindness and has affected more than 10,000 people in Japan. As clioquinol-zinc chelate is considered a mitochondrial toxin, it is one of the main causes of SMON. Furthermore, clioquinol could potently inhibit the 20S proteasome via Cu-dependent and Cu-independent mechanisms and consequently cause cell death due to the intracellular accumulation of misfolded proteins. Additionally, the discontinuation of clioquinol has been

P. Khan Mohammad Beigi, E. Maverakis,
Acrodermatitis Enteropathica: A Clinician's Guide,
DOI 10.1007/978-3-319-17819-6_6,
© Springer International Publishing Switzerland 2015

reported to lead to the elimination of SMON. Consequently, clioquinol was withdrawn from the market as an oral agent in the 1970s [2, 3].

Moynahan et al. discovered that AE is a zinc deficiency disorder and proposed a treatment with the prescription of zinc supplements. This treatment has proven to be effective, inexpensive, reliable, and non-toxic; as a result, it has become the main source of AE treatment during the last few decades [4].

Previously AE was treated with the administration of the antimicrobial agent diiodohydroxyquinoline (diodoquin) at a daily dosage of 200–300 mg. It was effective but it resulted in the incomplete remission of symptoms. Treatment with diodoquin also had side effects, such as abdominal pain, goiter appearance, hair loss, furunculosis due to iodine sensitivity, agranulocytosis, fever, chills, headache, peripheral neuropathy, optic neuritis, and optic nerve atrophy [2]. Prescription of diodoquin was the main AE treatment method until there were reports of complete clinical remission due to the addition of zinc supplements to the patient's diet in 1973. From then on, administration of zinc supplements has become the main treatment method of AE. Today, clinical cases of AE are often treated with the administration of a daily dose of zinc supplements: 1–2 mg/kg in children and 220 thrice daily in adults. It is crucial for the administered treatment to continue and for zinc levels to be checked twice per year [5]. Long term zinc supplementation in AE is necessary to prevent any recurrence. Zinc acetate, zinc gluconate, and zinc sulfate are a few examples of available zinc supplements that can be effective in the treatment of AE. In cases of severe zinc deficiency, intravenous administration of 20–10 mg zinc chloride is recommended.

During treatment with zinc supplementation, some symptoms are seen to improve even prior to normalization of serum zinc levels. For instance, diarrhea is usually stopped within 24 h, psychological disorders and problems are resolved within 1–2 days, skin lesions begin to improve within 24 h, severe skin infections are healed within 1 week, and growth of hair becomes normal within 3–4 weeks [6].

References

1. Dillaha CJ, Lorincz AL, Aavik OR. Acrodermatitis enteropathica: review of the literature and report of a case successfully treated with diodoquin. JAMA. 1953;152(6):509–12.
2. Arbiser JL, et al. Clioquinol-zinc chelate: a candidate causative agent of subacute myelo-optic neuropathy. Mol Med. 1998;4(10): 665.
3. Bareggi SR, Cornelli U. Clioquinol: review of its mechanisms of action and clinical uses in neurodegenerative disorders. CNS Neurosci Ther. 2012;18(1):41–6.
4. Moynahan EJ. Letter: acrodermatitis enteropathica: a lethal inherited human zinc-deficiency disorder. Lancet. 1974;2(7877): 399–400.
5. Moynahan E. Acrodermatitis enteropathica in two siblings treated with zinc sulphate supplements alone. Proc R Soc Med. 1975;68(5):276.
6. Puri N. A study of efficacy of oral zinc therapy for acrodermatitis enteropathica. Nasza Dermatolologia Online. 2013;4:162–6.

Part II
Review of the Roles
of Zinc in Metabolism

Chapter 7
Role of Zinc in Different Body Systems

Zinc plays multiple roles in metabolism, which can be classified into three major categories: catalytic, structural and regulatory functions [1, 2]. Zinc functions as a component of the catalytic site of various enzymes (termed metalloenzymes), which was first described by Keilin and Mann in 1939 after demonstrating that the enzyme carbonic anhydrase (an essential enzyme involved in the metabolism of carbon dioxide) requires zinc for proper catalytic function [3]. In the catalytic site of carbonic anhydrase, zinc was found to function as a Lewis acid by accepting a pair of electrons [3]. In a similar manner, zinc also is essential for the catalytic function of multiple other enzymes including alcohol dehydrogenase, matrix metalloproteinases, alkaline phosphatase and various RNA polymerases [4–6].

Zinc also serves a structural role in the setting of zinc finger proteins, in which the zinc ions stabilize the unique secondary folded structure known as the zinc finger motif and contribute to the function of these proteins [7]. Zinc finger proteins are among the most abundant proteins in eukaryotes and have a diverse array of functions including DNA binding, transcriptional activation and regulation of cell processes such as apoptosis [7]. Retinoic acid receptors and vitamin D receptors also belong to the zinc finger family of proteins [8]. Finally, zinc ions serve an important regulatory function in that they are able to bind zinc-dependant proteins,

P. Khan Mohammad Beigi, E. Maverakis,
Acrodermatitis Enteropathica: A Clinician's Guide,
DOI 10.1007/978-3-319-17819-6_7,
© Springer International Publishing Switzerland 2015

as occurs with zinc binding to the metal response element transcription factor (MTF) which regulates gene expression in response to the presence of metal ions and oxidative stress [9]. The importance of this transcription factor in eukaryotes is highlighted by the discovery that that a loss of function mutation of MTF in mice was shown to be lethal [10].

Some individuals obtain high levels of zinc through their dietary sources. Interestingly, if a patient with zinc deficiency disorder obtained adequate dietary zinc, general clinical symptoms could be prevented. According to observations, individuals with hereditary zinc disorders, such as AE, that obtain high zinc content through their daily diet are often in less danger of having any severe problems caused by the disorder.

In order to study the clinical effects of deficiency, animal studies are often carried out due to the rarity of zinc deficiency in the modern varied human diet. One of the notable symptoms of AE observed in both children and animals is thymic atrophy and an increased susceptibility to infections: production of thymocytes and T-cells is reduced significantly [11].

It is important to note that zinc requirements depend on the physiological status of individuals. Compared a regular adult, a pregnant woman would have higher zinc requirements. Given the role of zinc in protein synthesis and other transcriptional processes, it would be logical for events that are associated with high metabolic activity, such as growth, pregnancy, and lactation, to require increased amounts of zinc [12].

Neutrophils, peripheral blood monocytes, tissue macrophages and mast cells require a minimum amount of zinc to function properly. In addition, zinc plays an important role in the metabolism of essential fatty acids. In regards to wound healing, zinc is a required nutrient. Zinc deficient patients have a slow and ineffective wound healing process, which is seen to improve quickly when zinc supplements are added to their diet. It is believed that high consumption of zinc through the diet has no pharmacological effect unless the body's zinc levels are abnormal. Furthermore, role of zinc in treating dermatological disorders is controversial and the effect of this mineral on acne is being studied and some results have been obtained.

7.1   Biochemistry of Zinc Metabolism

Since 1934, zinc has been considered an essential mineral required for growth of mice and rats, while it was still not known as a required nutrient for humans [13]. Finally in 1974, zinc consumption of up to 15 mg per day for normal adults and up to 20–25 mg per day during pregnancy was recommended by nutritional counselors. It is important to note that the average daily diet consumed in the United States supplies approximately 12–15 mg of zinc for an individual. On average the human body contains 2–3 mg of zinc. This amount is almost half of the amount of iron present in the body and 10–20 times more than other elements such as copper, magnesium, and nickel [14].

In solution, zinc often becomes a cation with a charge of 2+ and it is very rare for the Zn^{2+} ion to oxidize further, which implies its stability. This stability is an important characteristic of zinc.

After its absorption by the intestine, zinc is transferred into blood vessels in different forms: albumin-zinc complex (60–70 %), globulin-zinc complex (10–20 %), transferrin (1–5 %), amino acid (5–10 %), and amino-globulin (less than 1 %). All body tissues contain zinc, but the highest levels are present in muscles, epidermis of skin, liver, kidney, bones, and prostate glands.

Zinc is also present in hair; however, after long term zinc deficiency levels measureably decline and increases in zinc consumption can significantly influence the zinc concentration of the hair. In patients who have been zinc deficient for a only a short time, the concentration of zinc in hair does not decline appreciably and thus is not reliable for accurate evaluation of zinc status of the body [15].

The presence of zinc in body is very important for proper function of many enzymes, such as metalloenzymes [16]. In 1940, Keilin and Mann found that zinc exists in carbonic anhydrase [3]. Moreover, roughly twenty metalloproteinase enzymes are associated with zinc [16].

Zinc also plays a role in bone physiology, especially during the growth and development of young individuals. It was observed that the concentration of zinc in bone is significantly higher than that of other tissues and zinc is considered to be an essential component of the calcified matrix [17].

7.2   Skin and Hair Physiology

Zinc is involved in essential functions of epidermal physiology, especially the keratinization process. Zinc is often found in the granular layer of the epidermis and its concentration in epidermis is six times greater than that in other dermal tissues. The three main functions of zinc in the keratinization process are catalysis, structural and regulatory. The catalytic roles of zinc involve its activation of metalloenzymes, such as RNA nucleotide transferases, RNA polymerase, alcohol dehydrogenase, and carbonic anhydrase. Zinc also has a key role in the formation of structural proteins. The regulatory role of zinc during keratinization includes regulating calmodulin, thyroid hormone binding, protein kinase C, and inositol phosphate synthesis. Calmodulin is responsible for the release of Ca^{2+} into the cytosol, where the presence of calcium is essential for the activation of epidermal transglutaminase, which is important for development of the keratinocyte. The protein kinase C, also calcium dependent, carries out the phosphorylation of proteins during keratinization. The regulation of calmodulin and protein kinase C is done by the thyroid hormone, and the inositol phosphate increases the level of calcium [18, 19].

Alopecia, dermatitis, and secondary skin infections are the major clinical manifestations of zinc deficiency disorder in humans and animals. Secondary infections are commonly caused by Candida albicans and gram-positive bacteria; while gram-negative infections are caused by Pseudomonas aeruginosa [20]. For example, the activity of the enzymes such as glutamate dehydrogenase and aminotransferase is significantly affected by zinc deficiency. Consequently, amino acid metabolism and protein synthesis, which is required for epidermal regeneration, is considerably diminished in individuals with zinc deficiency. Zinc supplements have been effective in the treatment of many of these zinc deficiency disorders. Furthermore, researchers have observed that the consumption of dietary zinc results in a measurable increase of zinc levels in the epidermal tissue within 72 h of ingestion.

The primary skin lesions, such as bullous pustular dermatitis and polymorphic bulbous vesiculobullous eruptions have been observed as one of the main symptoms that is common within patients who are diagnosed with severe zinc deficiency disorder [21]. A visible feature of these epidermal eruptions is that they have hollow-centered erythematous surfaces. The outbreaks are usually symmetric and often located around the mouth, nose, eyelids, and external ears. The hands, head, elbows, knees, thighs, and hips are also at risk of getting infected [22]. These outbreaks appear in the form of psoriasis on the hips and around the mouth, often in a mask-shaped distribution. Infected lesions may be covered with purulent crusts and have the appearance of impetigo. In addition, lesions on the fingers may appear similar to Acrodermatitis Hallopeau. Cases of stomatitis, glossitis, and vulvitis have also been reported in patients. Losses of hair, eyebrows, and eyelashes have also been noted: strands of hair appear pale and thin and are readily detached without any resistance. As a result, zinc deficiency has been linked with alopecia [23].

7.3 Gastrointestinal System and Other Organs

Gastrointestinal symptoms often appear early in the disease course, coinciding with the onset of the epidermal eruptions. Patients have reported to have had diarrhea three to six times per day with colorless stools and sometimes brown, frothy, greasy and foul-smelling. These symptoms could be as a result of impaired absorption of water and electrolytes in the large

intestine. Interestingly, the severity of the epidermal outbreaks and gastrointestinal symptoms are often similar. In
addition, gastric and peptic ulcers have been reported as well
as diabetes, stomatitis, bleeding of the gums, and nosebleeds
have also been reported. In addition, zinc deficiency patients
who suffer from stomach ulcers have also reported ulcer
healing problems, which can be a fatal condition [24, 25].

7.4   Neurological Development, Growth, and Mental Status

The concentration and distribution of zinc in the brain varies
with the stage of development the brain is in. Moderate deficiency of zinc has been recognized as one of the causes of
growth failure and hypogonadism in males. Zinc deficiency
greatly affects growth and development in children and adolescents. Furthermore, there have been reports of mental
retardation, growth failure, mental lethargy, loss of appetite,
emotional disorders, weight loss, continuous fatigue, and
depression in patients who have been diagnosed with zinc
deficiency. There have been reports of permanent mental
retardation, schizophrenia, permanent skin damage, dwarfism, and even fatality in untreated patients [26].

7.5   Central Nervous System

There are two pathways through which zinc can reach the
brain: brain barrier system and cerebrospinal fluid (CSF) that
is formed by plexus choroid [27]. It is interesting to note that
zinc primarily reaches the brain through the blood-brain barrier. The influx mechanism of zinc in the brain still remains
unclear; however, the high zinc concentration in the paren-
chymal cells compared to the extracellular fluid is indicative
of existence of an energy-dependent absorption in the neu-

rons and glial cells. Yet no specific transporter involved in this process has been identified to date [27].

The distribution of zinc in the central nervous system is uneven, with the most abundant quantity being in the forebrain, more specifically the hippocampus and cerebral neocortex. The male infant hippocampal zinc concentration has been observed to reach an equilibrium within the first 5 years of life [28]. The cerebral zinc concentration has been seen to gradually increase in young individuals while being constant in adults [27]. Quantitatively speaking, the hippocampal zinc concentration is much greater than those of other elements, including calcium and iron [29]. Other parts of the brain, such as the amygdala, substantia nigra, lenticular nucleus, and the thalamus, contain significant quantities of zinc [29].

7.6 Enzymes

The primary catalytic function of zinc involves interaction with metalloenzymes as a cofactor in order to activate them, which often occurs when the zinc cofactor binds and becomes part of the enzyme's active site. The presence of zinc is essential for the activation of these metalloenzymes [16]. These metalloenzymes, which include DNA polymerases, RNA nucleotide transferases, RNA polymerases, alcohol dehydrogenase, and carbonic anhydrase, have many important biochemical functions throughout the body; such as DNA replication and transcription, metabolism and catabolism of proteins, fats, and carbohydrates.

It has been discovered that the activity of zinc-dependent metalloenzymes is critically influenced by the amount of zinc present. For example, the activity of alkaline phosphatase, which is an active enzyme in the testes, intestine, bones, esophagus, stomach, and kidneys, is greatly affected by the reduction of zinc concentration in tissues; which in turn affects the functionality and performance of the associated tissues and/or organs [30].

7.7   Endocrine System

It appears that the presence of zinc may influence the function of hormones such insulin, ACTH, glucocorticoids, gastrin, growth hormone (GH), testosterone, androgen, prolactin, luteinizing hormone (LH), and follicle stimulating hormone (FSH). For instance, the plasma levels of GH and testosterone were significantly lower in zinc deficient rats compared to normal rats. Zinc deficiency often leads to gonadal growth impairment in sexually immature rat males. Moreover, the administration of GH in zinc deficient mice that have no pituitary glands had no effect on their growth rate; whereas growth rate was increased after the administration of zinc [31]. The effect of zinc on LH and FSH production and secretion will be discussed in Sect. 7.11.

7.8   Nucleic Acids

Zinc plays a fundamental role in the catabolism and biosynthesis of DNA and RNA, as it acts as a cofactor for DNA and RNA polymerases. In addition, zinc may be involved in sustaining the structure of polynucleotides [32].

7.9   Cell Development and Cell Cycles

Zinc deficiency can result in growth disorder and birth defect in newborns, which is due to the regulatory role zinc has in cell division and proliferation. Research has shown that zinc deficiency has adverse effects on majority of the stages of cell cycle. Zinc is considered essential for the progress of biochemical reactions of cells and progression of the cell cycle: passing from G1 phase to S (synthesis phase), from S phase to G2 phase, from the G2 phase to mitosis, and accurate chromosomal disjunction. This is because of the presence of zinc dependent molecules that are significantly involved in the phenomena of replication and/or transcription of DNA; these molecules include chromatin replication enzymes, transcription factors, and regulatory hormones [17, 33].

The amount and type of histone proteins in the nucleus is influenced by the presence of zinc. It was observed that the content and properties of histone was altered in the brain and liver of zinc deficient rats, reducing the transcriptional capacity of the chromatin [28]. Furthermore, enzymes such as DNA polymerase and RNA polymerase, which are respectively essential to replication and transcription, cannot function without the presence of zinc [34, 35]. There are also many transcription factors that are zinc dependent, like the finger transcription protein, WT-1, which is crucial for the development of kidney and gonads. During kidney development, WT-1 binds to the regulatory regions of some developmental genes and is believed to also prevent the expression of certain growth factors, such as insulin growth factor II (IGF-II) [36, 37]. Another zinc dependent transcription factor is Krox 20, which regulates the expression of the hindbrain development gene.

Furthermore, the presence of zinc is also essential for accurate chromosome segregation during meiosis. As a result, zinc deficiency may result in the production of defective or deficient gametes [38]. In addition, zinc deficiency is known as one of the causes of hypogonadism in males [31].

7.10   Reproduction System

Zinc is essential for the proper function of the cells of reproductive system such as sperm, oocytes, and embryonic cells. The differentiation and proliferation of these cells are highly dependent on zinc; as a result, they are highly sensitive to zinc deficiency. It has been reported that zinc deficiency caused reduction in pituitary gland and accessory sex organ size in male rats. It was observed that all the observed changes except testicular and epididymis atrophy were reversed when zinc was added to the diet [39]. This illustrates the importance of zinc in the development of the reproductive system.

7.11   Fertility Control

The high zinc concentration present in the reproductive system, including the prostate gland, the seminal fluid, and the ejaculate sperm, points to the possible role zinc may have in fertility, along with copper and selenium [28, 40]. Zinc has three main roles in the cells of reproduction system: developmental, morphological, and hormonal.

Zinc deficiency in humans has been associated with maturation delay of sex organs as well as decreased testicular response to pituitary secretion stimulation [41]. Zinc plays a role in the conversion of angiotensin during the production of testosterone by Leydig cells [40]. As a result, men with low cellular zinc concentrations have low levels of testosterone [42]; which suggests the significance of zinc for spermatogenesis. In addition, zinc is also involved in determining the motility and life span of these cells [43, 44]. It was also discovered that zinc regulates conversion of testosterone to other secondary sex neurohormones such as dihydrotestosterone. Hence, it appears that zinc supplementation is beneficial for male sterility [41].

Furthermore, zinc is involved in the synthesis and secretion of follicle stimulating hormone (FSH) and luteinizing hormone (LH). Consequently, zinc deficiency would cause abnormalities in the hormonal cycle resulting in irregular development of ovaries as well as menstrual cycle problems [40, 41]. Zinc deficiency could also have a significant effect on a pregnant individual as zinc requirements increase sharply during pregnancy [17]; hence it can result in spontaneous abortion, increased risk of hypertension and pre-eclampsia, or increased risk of neonatal morbidity. Lactation could also be greatly affected by zinc deficiency as low zinc concentration would prevent the normal activity of prolactin, which requires zinc for the stimulation of breast tissue development and milk production [28].

It was reported that zinc deficiency in pregnant rats resulted in slow early embryonic development, resulting in abnormalities of the cytoplasm and blastocoel cavity, decreased rate of embryonic resorption (ability of viable embryo to be implanted in the uterus wall), and increased risk of defective development of vital organs during fetal development, such as cranial bone and brain. Comparably, moderate zinc deficiency was been associated with delayed intrauterine growth [17].

7.12   Cell Membranes

Zinc is necessary for normal cell membrane functionality and stability. For example, zinc has inhibitory effects. Zinc prevents the induced release of histamine from mast cells; and it also prevents platelet aggregation. The mentioned functions are carried out through the binding of zinc to specific membrane receptors. It is important to note that there is an antagonistic relationship present between calcium and zinc regarding stimulation and/or stabilization of the cell membrane. For instance, cell activities that are inhibited by zinc are activated by calcium: calcium has stimulatory effects on the releasing of histamine from mast cells and platelet aggregation [45].

7.13   Synthesis of Proteins and Collagen

It has been shown that zinc is essential for protein metabolism and synthesis, and it is often prescribed to zinc deficient patients to help with wound healing. For example, amino acid uptake in the liver and chromosomal protein synthesis was observed to significantly decrease in zinc deficient rats compared to the control group [46]. The detrimental effect of zinc deficiency on nucleic acid and protein metabolism and synthesis is the cause of improper depositing of collagen in connective tissues of the body. Zinc deficiency impairs the proliferation of fibroblasts, therefore causing a reduction in collagen content, which results in wound healing problems in patients [47]. Furthermore, research showed that synthesis of nucleic acids and proteins become normal in zinc deficient rats after they were fed supplemental zinc [46].

7.14   Immune System

Zinc deficiency is a well-known cause of cell-mediated immunity dysfunction, which would leave the zinc deficient individual unprotected against fungal, viral, and pathogenic attacks [48]. It is important to note that zinc supplementation is observed to correct all immune defects that are caused by zinc deficiency. Immunological defects linked to zinc deficiency disorders include lymphopenia, depressed T-cell mitogenic response, increased numbers of circulating suppressor T-cells, and decreased natural killer activity. The reduction in the concentration of active thymulin in the plasma is known as one of the early effects of zinc deficiency in humans: thymulin induces the production of T-cells [49]. Furthermore, zinc deficiency is seen to impair immune system functions and reduce humoral and cellular responses which is caused by the reduction of lymphocytes and T cells. The bactericidal and phagocytic capacities of macrophages are also seen to diminish in the setting of zinc deficiency [50].

There has been interest in the idea that zinc supplementation may be able to correct loss of immunological responsivity associated with aging. Cellular immunity in the elderly has been observed to improve by the administration of zinc supplementation; but, further clarification of this proposition is needed [51, 52].

References

1. Maret W. Zinc and human disease. In: Interrelations between essential metal ions and human diseases. Dordrecht: Springer; 2013. p. 389–414.
2. Cousins RJ. Metal elements and gene expression. Annu Rev Nutr. 1994;14(1):449–69.
3. Keilin D, Mann T. Carbonic anhydrase. Purification and nature of the enzyme. Biochem J. 1940;34(8-9):1163.

4. Plocke DJ, Levinthal C, Vallee BL. Alkaline phosphatase of Escherichia coli: a zinc metalloenzyme*. Biochemistry. 1962;1(3):373–8.

5. Kagi J, VALLEE BL. The role of zinc in alcohol dehydrogenase. V. The effect of metal-binding agents on the structure of the yeast alcohol dehydrogenase molecule. J Biol Chem. 1960;235: 3188–92.

6. Scrutton M, Wu C, Goldthwait D. The presence and possible role of zinc in RNA polymerase obtained from Escherichia coli. Proc Natl Acad Sci. 1971;68(10):2497–501.

7. Laity JH, Lee BM, Wright PE. Zinc finger proteins: new insights into structural and functional diversity. Curr Opin Struct Biol. 2001;11(1):39–46.

8. Umesono K, et al. Direct repeats as selective response elements for the thyroid hormone, retinoic acid, and vitamin D_3 receptors. Cell. 1991;65(7):1255–66.

9. Daniels PJ, et al. Mammalian metal response element-binding transcription factor-1 functions as a zinc sensor in yeast, but not as a sensor of cadmium or oxidative stress. Nucleic Acids Res. 2002;30(14):3130–40.

10. Günes Ç, et al. Embryonic lethality and liver degeneration in mice lacking the metal-responsive transcriptional activator MTF-1. EMBO J. 1998;17(10):2846–54.

11. Fraker PJ, Gershwin ME, Good RA, Prasad A. Interrelationships between zinc and immune function. Fed Proc 1986;45:1474–9.

12. Krebs NF. Overview of zinc absorption and excretion in the human gastrointestinal tract. J Nutr. 2000;130(5):1374S–7.

13. Saper RB, Rash R. Zinc: an essential micronutrient. Am Fam Physician. 2009;79(9):768.

14. Sandstead HH. Zinc nutrition in the United States. Am J Clin Nutr. 1973;26(11):1251–60.

15. Van Wouwe JP. Clinical and laboratory assessment of zinc deficiency in Dutch children. A review. Biol Trace Elem Res. 1995;49(2-3):211–25.

16. Piperi C, Papavassiliou AG. Molecular mechanisms regulating matrix metalloproteinases. Curr Top Med Chem. 2012;12(10): 1095–112.

17. Salgueiro MJ, et al. The role of zinc in the growth and development of children. Nutrition. 2002;18(6):510–9.

18. Brewer GJ, et al. Zinc inhibition of calmodulin: a proposed molecular mechanism of zinc action on cellular functions. Am J Hematol. 1979;7(1):53–60.

19. Krebs J. Calmodulin-dependent protein kinase IV: regulation of function and expression. Biochimica et Biophysica Acta (BBA)-Molecular. Cell Res. 1998;1448(2):183–9.
20. Van Wouwe JP. Clinical and laboratory diagnosis of acrodermatitis enteropathica. Eur J Pediatr. 1989;149(1):2–8.
21. Kumar P, et al. Zinc and skin: a brief summary. Dermatol Online J. 2012;18(3):1.
22. Aggett PJ. Acrodermatitis enteropathica. J Inherit Metab Dis. 1983;6 Suppl 1:39–43.
23. Perafán-Riveros C, et al. Acrodermatitis enteropathica: case report and review of the literature. Pediatr Dermatol. 2002;19(5):426–31.
24. Watanabe T, et al. Zinc deficiency delays gastric ulcer healing in rats. Dig Dis Sci. 1995;40(6):1340–4.
25. McClain CJ, Su LC. Zinc deficiency in the alcoholic: a review. Alcohol Clin Exp Res. 1983;7(1):5–10.
26. Grønli O, et al. Zinc deficiency is common in several psychiatric disorders. PLoS One. 2013;8(12), e82793.
27. Takeda A. Zinc homeostasis and functions of zinc in the brain. Biometals. 2001;14(3-4):343–51.
28. Vallee BL, Falchuk KH. The biochemical basis of zinc physiology. Physiol Rev. 1993;73(1):79–118.
29. Tuormaa TE. Adverse effects of zinc deficiency: a review from the literature. J Orthomol Med. 1995;10:149–64.
30. Naber TH, et al. Serum alkaline phosphatase activity during zinc deficiency and long-term inflammatory stress. Clin Chim Acta. 1996;249(1):109–27.
31. Root AW, et al. Effects of zinc deficiency upon pituitary function in sexually mature and immature male rats. J Nutr. 1979;109(6):958–64.
32. Slater JP, Mildvan AS, Loeb LA. Zinc in DNA polymerases. Biochem Biophys Res Commun. 1971;44(1):37–43.
33. Falchuk KH, Montorzi M. Zinc physiology and biochemistry in oocytes and embryos. In: Zinc biochemistry, physiology, and homeostasis. London: Springer; 2001. p. 199–209.
34. Dreosti IE. Zinc and the gene. Mutat Res/Fundam Mol Mech Mutagen. 2001;475(1):161–7.
35. Prasad AS. Clinical, biochemical and nutritional spectrum of zinc deficiency in human subjects: an update. Nutr Rev. 1983;41(7): 197–208.
36. Drummond I, et al. Repression of the insulin-like growth factor II gene by the Wilms tumor suppressor WT1. Science. 1992;257(5070):674–8.

37. Werner H, et al. The regulation of IGF-I receptor gene expression. Int J Biochem Cell Biol. 1995;27(10):987–94.
38. Kumari D, Nair N, Bedwal RS. Effect of dietary zinc deficiency on testes of Wistar rats: morphometric and cell quantification studies. J Trace Elem Med Biol. 2011;25(1):47–53.
39. Millar M, et al. The effects of dietary zinc deficiency on the reproductive system of male rats. Can J Biochem Physiol. 1958;36(6):557–69.
40. Bedwal R, Bahuguna A. Zinc, copper and selenium in reproduction. Experientia. 1994;50(7):626–40.
41. Favier AE. The role of zinc in reproduction. Biol Trace Elem Res. 1992;32(1-3):363–82.
42. Prasad AS, et al. Zinc status and serum testosterone levels of healthy adults. Nutrition. 1996;12(5):344–8.
43. Andrews JC, et al. Role of zinc during hamster sperm capacitation. Biol Reprod. 1994;51(6):1238–47.
44. Henkel R, et al. Relevance of zinc in human sperm flagella and its relation to motility. Fertil Steril. 1999;71(6):1138–43.
45. Marone G, Findlay SR, Lichtenstein LM. Modulation of histamine release from human basophils in vitro by physiological concentrations of zinc. J Pharmacol Exp Therap. 1981;217(2):292–8.
46. Kimball SR, et al. Effects of zinc deficiency on protein synthesis and expression of specific mRNAs in rat liver. Metabolism. 1995;44(1):126–33.
47. SANDSTEAD HH, et al. Zinc and wound healing. Effects of zinc deficiency and zinc supplementation. Am J Clin Nut. 1970;23:514–9.
48. McMurray D. Cell-mediated immunity in nutritional deficiency. Prog Food Nutr Sci. 1983;8(3-4):193–228.
49. Prasad AS, et al. Serum thymulin in human zinc deficiency. J Clin Invest. 1988;82(4):1202.
50. Wirth J, Fraker P, Kierszenbaum F. Zinc requirement for macrophage function: effect of zinc deficiency on uptake and killing of a protozoan parasite. Immunology. 1989;68(1):114.
51. Shankar AH, Prasad AS. Zinc and immune function: the biological basis of altered resistance to infection. Am J Clin Nutr. 1998;68(2):447S–63.
52. Keen CL, Gershwin ME. Zinc deficiency and immune function. Annu Rev Nutr. 1990;10(1):415–31.

Part III
Cases Descriptions of
Acrodermatitis Enteropathica

Chapter 8
History of Acrodermatitis Enteropathica in Adults

In this report, we describe several cases of AE, which were observed around the patients' time of puberty. In 1952, Peeper reported the case of a 46-year-old woman, who had a mild form of AE; and her main symptom was diarrhea with mucoid stools. The patient's parents were third cousins and one of their siblings was reported to have had the symptoms of this disorder. Next, the case of a 23-year-old woman was described whose symptoms started when she was eight years old and her symptoms would only improve during her period of pregnancy [1].

In 1972, Guy reported the case of a 17-year-old boy who had the symptoms of epidermolysis bullosa which started when he was one years old and subsided in his maturity. The diagnosis was Acrodermatitis Enteropathica since both of his siblings were also diagnosed with AE [1].

Lastly, there was a case was of a 47-year-old Caucasian woman who suffered from advanced skin lesions which originated when she was three months old. As an infant, she was born naturally, weighed seven pounds, and was fed with infant formula. The parents of the patient were not blood-related and her family had no history of this disorder. She was previously hospitalized because of the same disorder and received oral steroid treatment; however, her disorder was not cured. The patient was unable to move or walk for six months due to the impairments caused by the disorder to her

P. Khan Mohammad Beigi, E. Maverakis,
Acrodermatitis Enteropathica: A Clinician's Guide,
DOI 10.1007/978-3-319-17819-6_8,
© Springer International Publishing Switzerland 2015

hands and feet. She also recalled the pain she felt in her childhood due to nail blisters. Furthermore, the greatest amount of skin damage was seen in the patient's gluteal area. Whenever the wounds and skin damages worsened, the patient's conditions worsened as well. The patient had dermatitis infections, but had healthy lungs. Severe loss of eyebrows, eyelashes, hair of groin and armpits were also seen in this patient. Other symptoms of this patient were blepharitis, stomatitis, glossitis, perleche, and conjunctivitis. The intake of bovine milk was reported to cause bloating and severe damage to the patient's skin but diarrhea and other gastrointestinal problems were not observed [1].

As mentioned in the introduction, AE has long been the subject of interest among dermatologists, pediatricians, and medical researchers. The disorder's primary stages, variant clinical forms, effects on different age groups, and treatment have been the center of discussion and research among doctors. At this time, in order to clarify the issue and examine it further, we will discuss and examine several cases reported in Iranian hospitals as well as academic journals.

Reference

1. Sardadvar S, Mostoufi M. Dermatology disorders. Tehran, Iran: Vol. 1. TUMS; 1972.

Chapter 9
Iranian Hospital Cases in Literature

9.1 Patient One [1]

This is the first Acrodermatitis Enteropathica patient in Iran that was reported by Dr. Sardadvar. This patient was a 6-month-old baby boy at the time of his admission to Razi Hospital on January 21, 1970. He was suffering from skin rash, digestion problems, and diarrhea. The patient had three brothers and two sisters who were apparently healthy. He had a natural birth, a normal weight at birth, and had been breast fed. The 6-year-old patient was suffering from a mild diarrhea at birth. Next, he had itching skin of the thighs, diarrhea, and hair loss at three months old. It is important to note that the history of the patient's disorder was intermittent and he did not respond to the administration of Mycostatin when he was 3 years old. The patient was re-admitted and examined at the age of 6 months old. The skin lesions still existed around the mouth, nose, eyes, hips, and anal canal. The lesions were in the form of squamous erythematous plaques that were restricted around the nose, mouth and chin and had spread to the anterior part of the neck. The recent lesions had red color that could be separated from normal skin because of its red areola, plaque centers slightly sunken, and cloudy content covered by a thin crust. Impetigo like lesions were seen in the inner angle of the eyes, on the jowl, and eyebrows. Red irregular plaques, which seemed like impetigo or eczema,

P. Khan Mohammad Beigi, E. Maverakis,
Acrodermatitis Enteropathica: A Clinician's Guide,
DOI 10.1007/978-3-319-17819-6_9,
© Springer International Publishing Switzerland 2015

were also observed in the area of head and neck. Skin eruption vesicles were seen on the fingers, hips and legs. Alopecia was also noticed on the head and eyebrows. In addition, his strands of hair were thin and pale, and the mucosa membrane of his nasal cavity and the mouth were red. The Patient also suffered from diarrhea and excretion was done five to six times per day. Stools were reported to be green or sometimes yellow, smelly, and mixed with white rashes.

The height and weight of the child were measured to be 88 cm and 9 kg respectively. He also suffered from severe photophobia and his other organs appeared normal during examination. The 6-month-old infant also had a mild fever. The course of treatment was initiated with three EnteroVioform tablets and Mycostatin ointment, vioform hydrocortisone, and hand washing with 2 % aqueous eosin solution. The treatment took a month and it was very successful. The biopsy hyperkeratosis results showed a bit of spongiosis on the epidermis but the skin appeared normal and candidiasis was not seen in the stool or skin.

9.2   Patient Two [1]

The second Acrodermatitis Enteropathica patient in Iran was reported by Dr. Mostoufi at Razi Hospital. The patient, who was a 20-month-old baby girl at the time, was admitted to the hospital because of skin rash, diarrhea and hair loss. She had a natural birth and had normal weight at birth. She had seven sisters and one brother, all of which seemed healthy. The child was breastfed. Skin eruptions appeared on the legs, wrists, and face, especially around her mouth. It was reported that her diarrhea with defecation of six times a day started 30 days after the skin rashes first appeared; and 3 months later her hair and eyebrows began to fall. When the patient was first admitted, erythematous squamous dermatoses was observed around the mouth, nose, and chin. The skin rash on her wrists had the form of bracelets which progressed to the backhand. Moreover, the internal and posterior parts of her thighs and pubic area were covered with rashes. The patient had mild photophobia, but her other organs seemed to function normally. She weighed 10 kg and her height was 75 cm. In addition, there wasn't any Candida fungus detected in the stool sample. Her blood test results were 4,200,000 red blood cells, 12,000 white blood cells, 53 lymphocytes, 2 monocytes, 6 eosinophils, and 39 polynuclear leukocytes. There were no specific symptoms detected in the skin biopsy since there was only a lack of keratinized stratified pitted cells in the epidermis. Furthermore, as the patient was diagnosed with Acrodermatitis Enteropathica upon clinical criteria. she was treated with four daily EnteroVioform tablets. Her symptoms significantly improved in the first week of her treatment.

Reference

1. Sardadvar S, Mostoufi M. Dermatology disorders. Tehran, Iran: Vol. 1. TUMS; 1972.

Chapter 10
Clinical Research Case Descriptions

10.1 Patient One

The patient was a 21-month old Caucasian boy with normal birth weight who had a history of acral lesions and periorificial dermatitis since he was 3 months old. He was breastfed until he was two and a half months old. He has a history of upper respiratory tract infections and otitis media which was treated in a private clinic. His parents were blood-related and his older brother, who had the same symptoms, had died at the age of 14 months. His preliminary skin examination showed plaque like scaly skin, erythematous, dry skin, and skin lesions on areas around the eyes, mouth, and diaper area. Additionally, there were reports of hair loss (alopecia), soft tissue infections around the nails (paronychia), and cracks and infection in the inguinal region. Physical examinations stated that the infant irritable and photophobic. His measured height and weight were 68 cm and 7.8 kg, respectively.

The infant patient was admitted to another hospital because of his chronic intermittent diarrhea, where his skin lesions were cured by the treatment of topical steroid and antifungal therapy. However, the disorder was not cured and the symptoms had not improved.

The patient was hospitalized at Razi Hospital when he was brought in for the evaluation of his skin lesions, which were caused by Staphylococcus aurous and septicemia caused by

P. Khan Mohammad Beigi, E. Maverakis,
Acrodermatitis Enteropathica: A Clinician's Guide,
DOI 10.1007/978-3-319-17819-6_10,
© Springer International Publishing Switzerland 2015

Klebsiella. He was treated with intravenous antibiotic therapy and after a few days his general condition improved, except for his skin lesions. The blood and urine tests were normal but his plasma zinc level was measured to be at 12 μg/dL (normal levels are 50–150 μg/dL). Moreover, microscopic examinations showed Candida albicans on the inguinal area, which was treated in 12 days by the administration of Baflokonazol 6 mg/kg/day. The patient was diagnosed with Acrodermatitis Enteropathica because of his clinical and laboratory test results. He was prescribed 40 mg of oral zinc sulfate per day which resulted in significant improvement of the symptoms within a few days, including the skin lesions. After a month of treatment, all lesions healed, hair began to grow back, and there were no reports of diarrhea. A follow up with the patient was recommended.

10.2   Patient Two

The patient was a 25-year-old woman. When she was 2 months old her mother stopped breastfeeding her and skin eruptions covered her entire body. The skin eruptions, such as vesiculobullous and erythematous scaly lesions, started around her mouth and spread throughout her face and legs. She also had diarrhea. Since she had symptoms suggestive of AE, there were further tests done in order to confirm the diagnosis. The diagnosis was confirmed by measurement of the plasma zinc levels which were at 0.2 mg/L (normal levels are between 0.7 and 1.6 mg/L). Her treatment began with administration of four tablets of 40 mg zinc sulfate per day. After 4 days, there was incredible improvement of her skin rashes and diarrhea, but she had developed behavior disorders. During these 25 years she continued her zinc supplementation treatment.

When she was 15 years of age, her treatment was reduced from 220 mg three times daily to twice daily. However, after 2 weeks, skin lesions began to appear around the mouth. When she was 16 she developed severe vomiting; and as a result, her treatment was increased to 220 mg of spansule-zinc supplements three times a day again. Afterwards, her plasma zinc was decreased from 1.1 to 0.3 mg/L and she suffered from rashes, similar to eczema and mild seborrheic dermatitis, on the sides of her nose and rashes similar to acne on her body. These rashes began to disappear 3 weeks after the increasing of spansule-zinc supplements to three times a day: plasma zinc increased to 1 mg/L.

Plasma zinc levels were measured at regular intervals of 6 months. When the patient reached the age of 20, her plasma zinc level decreased to the lowest normal level: 0.7 mg/L. The spnasule-zinc treatment was increased to 10 times a day. Fortunately, the patient's body was able to tolerate 10 pills per day and her plasma zinc level was maintained at a normal level of 1.4 mg/L.

Since this medication was not supported by the NHS, the patient had to pay the entire cost of her treatment for a long time. She used Oral Contraceptive Pills (Brevinor) without any effects on AE: OCP has been known as one of the causes of zinc deficiency. In addition the minor increase in zinc demand by the patient's body is because of fetal development. As a result, when the patient was pregnant, the level of plasma zinc was kept constant, since this deficiency disorder may be teratogenic. It is important for plasma zinc levels to be maintained at a normal concentration, because zinc deficiency may result in behavior and mood disorders, such as Cerebellar disorders, Parkinsonism, and cortical atrophy.

10.3   Patient Three

The patient was a 10-month-old female baby when she was administer to Razi Hospital, who presented skin eruptions, including sharply demarcated patches of vesiculobullous dermatitis on the cheeks, fingers, and in the diaper region when she was 2 months old. Her initial skin manifestations appeared 2 weeks after her weaning. She also showed symptoms of recurrent diarrhea, partial alopecia, and growth retardation. She was also observed to be irritable and had photophobia.

It is interesting to note that the patient's parents were not blood-relatives. The patient was born by a full term normal delivery; however since she had symptoms suggestive of AE, there were further tests done in order to confirm the diagnosis. Liver and renal function test results were normal. The diagnosis was confirmed by measurement of the serum zinc levels which were at 35 µg/dL (normal levels are between 70 and 150 µg/dL). Her serum alkaline phosphatase levels were also low at 57 IUL (normal levels are between 115 and 360 IUL).

The patient began substitution therapy with zinc sulfate 5 mg/kg body weight (50 mg daily) which led to the cessation of diarrhea after 2 weeks. The patient's plasma zinc levels were measured at regular intervals of 6 months. During the patient's follow- up after 4 months, the infant exhibited normal development and there was no recurrence of lesions or diarrhea.

10.4   Patient Four

This patient was a 4-month-old female baby when she was administered to Razi Hospital, who presented multiple well-defined erythematous, oozy crusted lesions on hands, feet, and periorificial areas. She developed these lesions 1 month after weaning. She was born by full term normal delivery to non-consanguineous parents. After further clinical examinations it was reported that she had normal anthropometric measurements, but was irritable. Furthermore, there was no report or indication of diarrhea or photophobia.

Since she had symptoms suggestive of AE, there were further tests done in order to confirm the diagnosis. Hematogram, liver, and renal function test results were normal; however, her serum zinc levels were at 48 µg/dL (normal levels are between 70 and 150 µg/dL). Her serum alkaline phosphatase levels were normal at 213 IUL (normal levels are between 115 and 360 IUL).

One week after the administration of zinc sulfate 5 mg/kg body weight (50 mg daily) the cutaneous lesions showed signs of improvement. One month after the administration, her serum zinc level was re-measured and the level was found to be higher at 102 µg/dL. During discharge, lifelong continuation of oral zinc supplementation was advised.

10.5   Patient Five

A 9-month-old male baby was administered to Razi Hospital after visiting the local clinic with superinfected, sharply demarcated, symmetrical erythematous macules and vesicles. Yellow-coloured crust manifestations were observed on the patient's cheeks as well as on the perioral, perianal, fingers, and diaper region. The baby was born by full term normal delivery and his parents were second degree blood-relatives. The skin lesions had appeared 1 week after weaning and he also showed signs of irritability and photophobia.

The infant's 4-year-old sister was also reported to be affected by similar manifestations and so the initial diagnosis of the clinic physician was a contagious impetigo. However, the suspected contagious impetigo had failed to respond to both topical and systemic antibiotics. Further clinical and laboratory tests were done at Razi hospital. Hematogram, liver, and renal function test results were normal; however, his serum zinc level was at 35 µg/dL (normal levels are between 70 and 150 µg/dL). His serum alkaline phosphatase levels were at 87 IUL (normal levels are between 115 and 360 IUL).

The patient was administered zinc sulfate 5 mg/kg body weight (60 mg daily). After 2 weeks of administration, the skin lesions showed signs of improvement. It was observed that his serum zinc level was found to be higher at 116 µg/dL, when measured 1 month later. Lastly, during discharge, lifelong continuation of oral zinc supplementation was advised.

10.6   Patient Six

A 4-year-old girl, sister of patient five that was described in the previous section presented similar lesions localized on her face, hands, and body folds. She was administered to Razi Hospital after the suspected impetigo failed to respond to both topical and systemic antibiotics. Dermatological examinations revealed eroded and beige coloured dry patches on the dorsum of the hands, perioral, and inguinal regions. As it was mentioned previously, the girl's parents were second degree blood-relatives.

Further clinical and laboratory tests were done at Razi hospital. Her serum zinc level was measured at 63 μg/dL (normal levels are between 70 and 150 μg/dL) and her serum alkaline phosphatase levels were measured at 280 IUL (normal levels are between 115 and 360 IUL).

The patient was administered zinc sulfate 5 mg/kg body weight, and 2 week later the skin lesions showed signs of improvement.

10.7   Patient Seven

The patient was a 2-month-old male baby, who was administered to Razi Hospital. He presented perioral and acral bullous lesions: the acral sites being the patient's hands and feet. These manifestations were variable sized vesicles and pustules with an erythematous base. The patient was observed to be febrile and irritable. There were no reports or indications of diarrhea or photophobia. He was born by full term normal delivery and was breast fed. The skin lesions appeared two weak after weaning. There was no family history of zinc deficiency.

Since he had symptoms suggestive of AE, there were further tests done in order to confirm the diagnosis. Hematogram, liver, and renal function test results were normal; however, his serum zinc levels were at 43 μg/dL (normal levels are between 70 and 150 μg/dL). This test result was used to confirm the AE diagnosis. His serum alkaline phosphatase levels were normal at 180 IUL (normal levels are between 115 and 360 IUL).

The patient was administered zinc sulfate 5 mg/kg body weight (50 mg daily). After 2 weeks of administration, the skin lesions showed signs of improvement. It was observed that his serum zinc level was improved to 103 μg/dL, when measured 1 month later.

10.8 Zinc Deficiency Similarities to AE in Infants (Eighth Patient)

The patient was a 15-week-old infant with the symptoms of skin rash, loss of appetite, and diarrhea. The skin rash did not respond to topical steroid treatment, antibiotics, antifungal, or protective creams. The patient was born prematurely at 35 weeks with normal skin. His parents were not blood-related and his growth chart was normal. From birth he was exclusively breastfed, and his parents did not report any history of specific disease or disorders. Additionally, the patient's sibling was reported to be healthy and had no history of skin disease. The examinations showed psoriasiform plaques in the groin and peripheral scaling. There were also circular patches observed on both of his cheeks and lips. Dark red psoriasiform plaques were also spotted on the surface of occipital in the posterior hairline, similar to the rashes present around the eyes and mouth. Furthermore, the patient was diagnosed with zinc deficiency since his plasma levels of zinc were at 3 µg/L (normal range is 11–24 µg/L). Oral zinc treatment (22.5 mg/day) resulted in rapid, successful improvements in symptoms: patient's appetite, dermatitis on his chest, other skin eruption, and diarrhea were all showing signs of improvement within 5 days of treatment. This case is suggestive of a transient form of zinc deficiency in and not hereditary AE.

Part IV
Acrodermatitis Enteropathica
Clinical Research

Chapter 11
Acrodermatitis Enteropathica

11.1 Synopsis of Study

AE (Acrodermatitis Enteropathica) is an autosomal recessive disorder affecting the uptake of zinc which causes reduction of all body zinc levels, including blood serum. Similar symptoms of severe zinc deficiency have often been observed in patients who underwent a prolonged intravenous nutrition. Common symptoms of AE include the appearance of perleche, skin lesions, erythematous patches, plaques of dry and scaly skin, and eczematous plaques on the face, scalp, and genital area. It is interesting to note that AE was frequently observed in Europe, particularly Northern Europe; and cases of AE have also been reported every year in Iran since 1970. AE is considered a minor and treatable disorder as long as it is diagnosed and treated promptly. It can be treated by supplementing the patient's diet with necessary amounts of zinc which would raise the level of zinc in blood plasma to normal levels.

Being a recessive autosomal disorder, which presents clinical symptoms if an individual of any gender is homozygous for the disease-related-gene, AE has become more common in Iran since it was first reported in 1970. It is interesting to note that Iran contains high numbers of consanguineous marriage especially in rural areas and tribes. Furthermore, malnutrition and dietary zinc deficiency contribute to the manifestation and severity of the clinical symptoms of this disorder. Many rural populaces of Iran are reported to have

P. Khan Mohammad Beigi, E. Maverakis,
Acrodermatitis Enteropathica: A Clinician's Guide,
DOI 10.1007/978-3-319-17819-6_11,
© Springer International Publishing Switzerland 2015

malnutrition, particularly neonatal and school-aged childhood. As a result, number of reported AE cases has been increasing in Iran. Therefore, conducting more research studies on this disorder and its complications is of great significance, especially in a country like Iran. The opportunity of conducting various studies in this field seems endless. AE has rarely been studied which may be due to the very few number of diagnosed and reported cases. The disorder is occasionally reported in patients who have been hospitalized for a long time and undergo intravenous nutrition.

With regards to the complications of AE, such as cutaneous, trichological, as well as neurological disorders, which are presented by reference texts and articles, further research studies are required to endorse or reject the symptoms and conditions as well as provide further information about AE. The present study has carried out by using the files of AE patients that were referred to Razi Hospital during the years 1999 to 2004.

11.2   Purpose of Study

The purpose of the study was to determine blood zinc levels and the symptoms of patients with Acrodermatitis Enteropathica, who were referred to Razi Hospital during the years 1999 to 2004. More specifically, the study aimed to determine the range of blood zinc levels of the mentioned patients as some AE cases have been reported to have normal blood zinc levels. Furthermore, the relationship between blood zinc level and the disorder's complications was investigated as well.

Alternate purposes:

- Indicate the relationship between blood zinc level and gastrointestinal symptoms in AE patients[1]
- Indicate the relationship between blood zinc level and alopecia in AE patients[2]

---

[1]Refers to any kind of ailment like gastrointestinal disorders or any alterations in

digestive system functions in the under study patients.

[2]Refers to excessive hair loss in any part of the body.

- Indicate the relationship between blood zinc level and cutaneous symptoms in AE patients[3]
- Indicate the relationship between blood zinc level and psychological symptoms in AE patients[4]

11.3   The Considered Hypotheses

1. Blood zinc level is less than normal in majority of AE patients.
2. There are some patients diagnosed with AE, whose blood zinc levels are normal.
3. Hair zinc level is less than normal in majority of AE patients.
4. Most AE patients suffer from gastrointestinal disorders (diarrhea, vomiting, and cramps).
5. The lower the blood zinc level is, the more serious the AE symptoms are.
6. All AE patients demonstrate cutaneous manifestations.
7. Most AE patients show psychological disorders such as moodiness, lethargy, anorexia, and photophobia.
8. The first symptom of the disorder is mucocutaneous lesions in most AE patients.
9. The first sign of recovery in most AE patients is the disappearance of cutaneous manifestations.
10. Most cases that are fed breast milk show the symptoms of the disorder as soon as they discontinue it.
11. Majority of the AE patients suffer from iron deficiency anemia and their blood ferritin and alkaline phosphatase levels are below normal.
12. There may be a correlation between zinc levels and iron levels if patients are iron deficiency anemia and blood ferritin and alkaline phosphatase levels return to normal by the prescription of zinc supplementation.

---

[3]Refers to any cutaneous manifestation such as acne, verrucose, eczema and other cutaneous disorders.
[4]Refers to any kind of psychological or mental disorders observable by the doctor.

11.4   Introduction

Being a recessive autosomal disorder, which presents clinical symptoms if an individual of any gender is homozygous for the disease-related-gene, Acrodermatitis Enteropathica has become more common in Iran since it was first reported in 1970. It is interesting to note that Iran contains high numbers of consanguineous marriage especially in rural areas and tribes. Furthermore, malnutrition and dietary zinc deficiency contribute to the manifestation and severity of the clinical symptoms of this disorder. Many rural populaces of Iran are reported to have malnutrition, particularly neonatal and school-aged childhood. As a result, number of reported AE cases has been increasing in Iran. Therefore, conducting more research studies on this disorder and its complications is of great significance, especially in a country like Iran.

The main purpose of the study was to determine blood zinc levels and the symptoms of 27 infant patients with Acrodermatitis Enteropathica, who were referred to Razi Hospital in Tehran, Iran during the years 1999 to 2004. More specifically, the study aimed to determine the range of blood zinc levels of the mentioned patients as some AE cases have been reported to possess normal serum zinc levels.

Furthermore, the secondary purpose of this study was to determine the relationship between blood zinc levels and the appearance and severity of symptoms, such as gastrointestinal symptoms, alopecia, cutaneous and psychological symptoms in AE patients.

11.5   Methods

The article is presented as a retrospective cross sectional study. Patients who had referred to the Razi Hospital Clinic or were sent to Razi Hospital by other medical clinics during 1999 to 2004 because of Acrodermatitis Enteropathica were considered and examined in this study: 27 infant patient cases were examined, of which 11 were male and 16 were female.

The location of study was at Razi Hospital's Dermatology Section located on Vahdat Eslami St. Tehran, Iran.

The study was also carried out by referring to the medial records of the considered patients that were available in the hospital archives. In cases where there was inadequate patient information available in the hospital archives or more information was needed, the patient was contacted and besides to ordering appropriate tests, an interview was set with the parents of the patient in order to complete the medical documents. Patients who were either not available and had incomplete hospital records or did not give their consent to be included in the clinical research were excluded from the study.

In order to obtain the zinc blood levels of the patients the following procedure was carried out. The blood sample was collected early in the morning since the normal circadian variation in plasma zinc levels is at its lowest and most precise during early mornings. The patients' parents were also told that their infant should be fasting before the blood test so that the test results would be accurate.

Furthermore, the patient medical records were used in order to complete the survey tool and patients were asked to come in for an interview if any further information was required or if there were questions that could not be answered based on the data from the medical documents. Geographically speaking, the patients were from many different parts of the country, such as Meshkin City, Kermanshah, Ghazvin, Marand, Ghaem City, Zanjan, Tehran, Boushehr, Shiraz, Tonekabon, and Fouman. Table 11.1 illustrates the types of variables that were measured in this study including a brief description about each one.

11.6   Ethical Considerations

- After filling out the survey tools, all medical files were returned to their former place and kept confidentially.
- The medical files were handled with care so that the documents were not physically damaged and all pages were kept intact.
- All Helsinki requirements were taken into account.

TABLE 11.1 Types of the measured variables

Row	Name of variable	Type of variable	Nominal or comparative/ continuous or discrete	Dependent or independent	Description	scale
1	Age	Quantitative (discrete)	Discrete	Independent	Patient's age is stated based on the month and the year of birth	Year
2	Weight	Quantitative (continuous)	Continuous	Independent	Patient's weight is stated based on kg	Kilogram
3	Sex	Qualitative (nominal)	Nominal	Independent	Patient's sex	Male/female
4	Place of birth	Qualitative (nominal)	Nominal	Independent	Place of birth is stated based on the name of the city and the state	City name
5	Father's age	Quantitative (discrete)	Discrete	Independent	Father's age is stated based on the year of birth	Year

6	Mother's age	Quantitative (discrete)	Discrete	Independent	Mother's age is stated based on the year of birth	Year
7	Parent's relationship	Qualitative (nominal)	Nominal	Independent	Parent's relativity is first degree, second degree or without relativity	First degree/second degree/no relativity
8	Cutaneous lesions	Qualitative (nominal)	Nominal	Dependent	The lesions are eczematous and erythematous, with scales around areas like the nose, eyes, genital and rectal areas	Around lips/nose/eyes/ Genital/rectal/fingers/ toes/elbow/hands/ foots/knee
9	Extremities cutaneous lesions	Qualitative (nominal)	Nominal	Dependent	Extremities lesions are eczematous and observed on fingers, toes, back of hands and foots, elbow, and knee	

(continued)

TABLE 11.1 (continued)

Row	Name of variable	Type of variable	Nominal or comparative/ continuous or discrete	Dependent or independent	Description	scale
10	Gastrointestinal Symptoms	Qualitative (nominal)	Nominal	Dependent	Any signs of diarrhea, vomiting, nausea, stomach ache or cramps are known as gastrointestinal signs	Diarrhea/vomiting/ stomach ache
11	Hair loss	Qualitative (nominal)	Nominal	Dependent	Hair loss is focal or diffused in any part of the body	Focal/ diffused
12	Neurologic symptoms	Qualitative (nominal)	Nominal	Dependent	Any sign of fatigue, moodiness, irritability, photophobia, or anorexia is known as neurologic symptoms	Lethargy/moodiness/ irritability/photophobia/ anorexia

13	Nail lesions	Qualitative (nominal)	Nominal	Dependent	Nail inflammatory lesions and nail border soft tissue inflammatory lesions are called parenchymal lesions	Nail plate/parenchymal
14	Onset of disorder	Quantitative (discrete)	Discrete	Dependent	The onset of disorder is stated as the number of months since the onset	Before and after weaning
15	Nutrition	Qualitative (nominal)	Nominal	Independent	Refers to the infant's nutrition which is mother's milk or cow's milk	Breastfeeding/ cow's milk
16	First symptoms	Qualitative (nominal)	Nominal	Dependent	The first symptom may be mucocutaneous gastrointestinal lesions, alopecia, or neurological/mental symptoms	Mucocutaneous lesions/ gastrointestinal lesions/ hair loss/neurological symptoms

(continued)

TABLE 11.1 (continued)

Row	Name of variable	Type of variable	Nominal or comparative/ continuous or discrete	Dependent or independent	Description	scale
17	Secondary mucocutaneous lesions	Qualitative (nominal)	Nominal	Dependent	Secondary cutaneous lesion in form of bacterial, viral, or candidal infections	Bacterial/viral/candidal infections
18	CBC	Quantitative (continuous)	Continuous	Dependent	CBC refers to the levels of WBCs and RBCs with platelets and Hb	Anemia/normal/ leukocytosis
19	Serum iron	Quantitative (continuous)	Continuous	Dependent	Refers to iron level in serum which is represented as µg/dL	µg/dL
20	Serum zinc level	Quantitative (continuous)	Continuous	Independent	Refers to zinc level in serum which is represented as µg/dL	µg/dL
21	Serum ferritin	Quantitative (continuous)	Continuous	Dependent	Refers to ferritin level in serum represented as µg/dL	µg/dL

| 22 | Amount of supplemental zinc | Quantitative (discrete) | Discrete | Refers to the amount of zinc prescribed to treat the patients, which is represented as mg/kg | mg/kg |
| 23 | First sign of recovery | Qualitative (nominal) | Nominal | The first sign of recovery may be identified as gastrointestinal lesions, mucocutaneous lesions, temperament, or recovery of hair loss | gastrointestinal/ cutaneous/mucoid/ neurological/alopecia |

11.7   Results

This study assessed patients clinically diagnosed with AE who presented to Razi Hospital during the years 1999 to 2004. A total of 27 infants were diagnosed with AE, whose information was obtained from their medical files or if required by contacting and re-examining them. As shown in Table 11.2, the average age of the patients was 8.9 months, ranging from 20 days to 5 years old. The average onset time of the disease was 37 days after birth, ranging from the 5th and 120th day from birth. The minimum ages of fathers and mothers were 22 and 18, respectively, and the maximum ages were 44 and 35, respectively, while the average ages were 31 and 25 years, respectively. The average patient weight was 6.5 kg, ranging from 3.2 to 10 kg. The minimum amount of serum zinc level was measured at 23 µg/dL and the maximum amount of it was 70 µg/dL, while the average amount was reported as 45.3 µg/dL. Table 11.3 illustrates that the surveyed patients were composed of 11 females (40.7 %) and 16 males (59.3 %). As seen in Table 11.4, 19 patients (70.4 %) had parents with first-degree blood-relativity and 5 patients

TABLE 11.2 Minimum, maximum, and mean values of Acrodermatitis Enteropathica patients' information who were admitted to Razi Hospital between 1999 and 2004

Categories	Minimum value	Maximum value	Mean value
Patient age (months)	0.7	60	8.9
Disorder start time (days from birth)	5	120	37.8
Patient weight (kg)	3.2	10	6.5
Father's age (years)	22	44	31.78
Mother's age (years)	18	35	25.37
Serum zinc content (µg/dL)	23	70	45.30

TABLE 11.3 Gender of Acrodermatitis Enteropathica patients admitted to Razi Hospital between 1999 and 2004

	Female		Male	
	Number of patients	**Percentage of patients**	**Number of patients**	**Percentage of patients**
Surveyed patients	11	40.7	16	59.3

TABLE 11.4 Acrodermatitis Enteropathica patients admitted to Razi Hospital between 1999 and 2004

	First degree blood-related[a]		Second degree blood-related[b]		Not blood-related	
	Number of Patients	**Percentage of Patients**	**Number of Patients**	**Percentage of Patients**	**Number of Patients**	**Percentage of Patients**
Surveyed patients	19	70.4	5	18.5 %	3	11.1

[a]A first degree blood-relative is defined as a blood relative which includes the individual's first-cousins
[b]A second degree blood-relative is defined as a blood relative which includes the individual's second-cousins

(18.5 %) had parents with second-degree blood-relativity, whereas in three cases (11.1 %) the parents were not related.

After the survey tools were completed, the data was transferred to SPSS software for analysis via the Mann-Whitney statistical test. The perioral, perinasal, perigenital, and perirectal lesions showed significant correlation with the level of serum zinc with the respective p-values of 0.006, 0.005, 0.005, and 0.008. On the other hands, periorbital lesions had no significant correlation with serum zinc levels: p-value = 0.139. Table 11.5 illustrates the extent of skin manifestations in the patients. Acral lesions and lesions on fingers, hands, elbow and feet also demonstrated significant correlation with patient serum zinc levels, with the respective p-values of 0.001, 0.003, 0.003, and 0.006. However, the lesions on toes, with p-value of 0.175, and knees, p-value = 0.4, had no significant correlation with serum zinc levels. Table 11.6

TABLE 11.5 Extent and site of skin manifestations of Acrodermatitis Enteropathica patients admitted to Razi Hospital between 1999 and 2004

	Present		Absent	
	Number of patients	Percentage of patients	Number of patients	Percentage of patients
Perioral manifestations	26	96.3	1	3.7
Prenasal manifestations	24	88.9	3	11.1
Periorbital manifestations	7	25.9	20	74.1
Perigenital manifestations	22	81.5	5	18.5
Perianal manifestations	19	70.4	8	29.6

TABLE 11.6 Extent and site of skin infections and eczematous skin lesions of Acrodermatitis Enteropathica patients admitted to Razi Hospital between 1999 and 2004

Manifestation Location	Present		Absent	
	Number of patients	Percentage of patients	Number of patients	Percentage of patients
Fingers	14	51.9	13	48.1
Toes	8	29.6	19	70.4
Back of hands	21	77.8	6	22.2
Back of legs	14	51.9	13	48.5
Ankles	17	63	10	37
Knees	18	66.7	9	33.3

shows the magnitude of skin infections and lesions among the patients. In regards to gastrointestinal symptoms, diarrhea and stomach ache symptoms were significantly correlated with the serum zinc levels with p-values of 0.001 and 0.008,

TABLE 11.7 Extent and magnitude of gastrointestinal symptoms of Acrodermatitis Enteropathica patients admitted to Razi Hospital between 1999 and 2004

	Present		Absent	
	Number of patients	Percentage of patients	Number of patients	Percentage of patients
Diarrhea	19	70.4	8	29.6
Vomiting	9	33.3	18	66.7
Stomach ache	14	51.9	13	48.1

TABLE 11.8 Extent and modes of hair loss (Alopecia) of Acrodermatitis Enteropathica patients admitted to Razi Hospital between 1999 and 2004

	Present		Absent	
	Number of Patients	Percentage of Patients	Number of Patients	Percentage of Patients
Focal	7	25.9	20	74.1
Diffusion	12	44.4	15	55.6

respectively; however, vomiting had no significant relation with it with a p-value of 0.4. It is important to note that since diarrhea is usually simultaneous with cramps, these two symptoms were observed concurrently. Moreover, Table 11.7 demonstrates the extent of gastrointestinal symptoms among patients. Table 11.8 illustrates the extent and mode of hair loss (Alopecia) in the AE patients. In addition to the statistics of the symptom, only diffused alopecia was significantly correlated with serum zinc levels. In regards to neurological symptoms, it was determined that fatigue, moodiness, irritability, photophobia, and anorexia are all significantly related to the serum zinc levels: the calculated respective p-values are 0.003, 0.008, 0.001, 0.004 and 0.003. Table 11.9 shows the extent of appearance of these symptoms in the patients. Furthermore, infants who were fed breast milk and presented AE symptoms after weaning demonstrated significant

TABLE 11.9 Extent and types of neurological symptoms of Acrodermatitis Enteropathica patients admitted to Razi Hospital between 1999 and 2004

Neurological Symptoms	Present		Absent	
	Number of Patients	Percentage of Patients	Number of Patients	Percentage of Patients
Fatigue	15	55.6	12	44.4
Moodiness	15	55.6	12	44.4
Irritability	15	55.6	12	44.4
Photophobia	11	40.7	16	59.3
Anorexia	26	96.3	1	3.7

correlation between the extent and magnitude of symptoms and serum zinc levels: p-value was 0.004. Infants that were fed infant formula or bovine milk and as a result presented symptoms also showed significant correlation between the extent and magnitude of symptoms and serum zinc levels: p-value was 0.001. Finally, with regards to the first symptom of the disorder, only the mucocutaneous manifestations were significantly related to serum zinc levels (p-value = 0.004); and with respect to the first sign of recovery, mucocutaneous manifestations illustrated significant correlation with serum zinc levels with the p-value being 0.004.

11.8   Discussion

According to the information obtained in this study, the cases were composed of 11 female (41 %) and 16 male (59 %) infants. Other studies have also provided evidence that the Acrodermatitis Enteropathica disorder is not sex-linked. All examined patients were at the neonatal period of infancy, which most credible references have related the disorder to this period of life. However, there have been very rare cases of the disorder reported in adults, even though these reports are not reported in this article.

Of the 27 patients surveyed, 25 of them had consanguineous parents while the other two patients' parents were not blood-related. Regarding the parents' relativity, it should be stated that 70.4 % of the cases (19 patients) had parents with first degree blood-relativity. In the case of the periorificial manifestations, 26 patients (96.3 %) had perioral manifestations, 24 cases (88.9 %) showed perinasal manifestations, 7 individuals (25.9 %) had periorbital manifestations, 22 patients (81.5 %) had perigenital manifestations, and 19 cases (70.4 %) were had perirectal manifestations. Our examinations revealed that 14 cases (51.9 %) had lesions on fingers, 8 (29.6 %) had toe lesions, and 21 (77.8 %) and 14 (51.9 %) showed lesions on back of hands and feet, respectively. Furthermore, 17 patients (63 %) had lesions on their elbows and 18 (66.7 %) on the knees.

All in all, Acrodermatitis Enteropathica is considered a severely fatal condition for infants if not diagnosed and treated promptly. It is vital for physicians all over the world to be alert about this disorder and its specific symptoms, especially in third world countries where consanguineous marriage is commonplace so that patients may be appropriately counseled regarding the risk of this and other autosomal recessive disorders to increase the recognition and early treatment of this treatable but potentially devastating disease.

Chapter 12
Case Photos

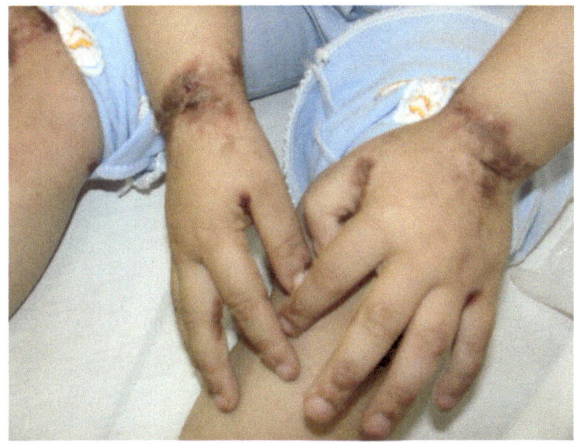

FIGURE 12.1 Hand and finger lesions (Source: Dr. P. Khan Mohammad Beigi, M.D.)

P. Khan Mohammad Beigi, E. Maverakis,
Acrodermatitis Enteropathica: A Clinician's Guide,
DOI 10.1007/978-3-319-17819-6_12,
© Springer International Publishing Switzerland 2015

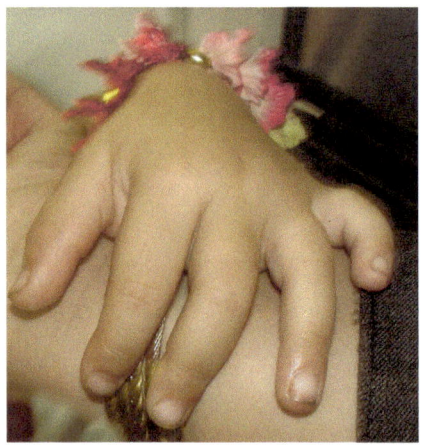

FIGURE 12.2 After treatment (healing of lesions) (Source: Dr. P. Khan Mohammad Beigi, M.D.)

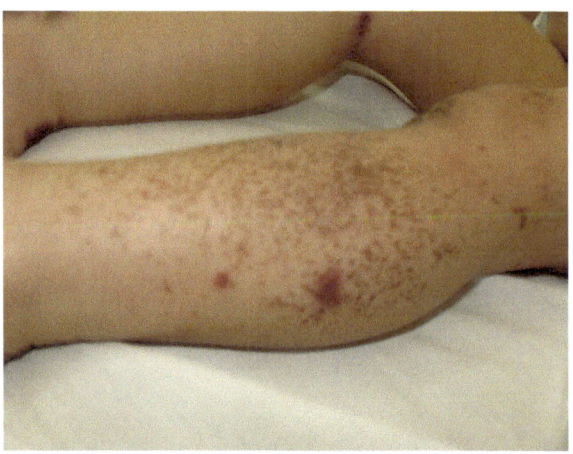

FIGURE 12.3 Lesions on legs (Source: Dr. P. Khan Mohammad Beigi, M.D.)

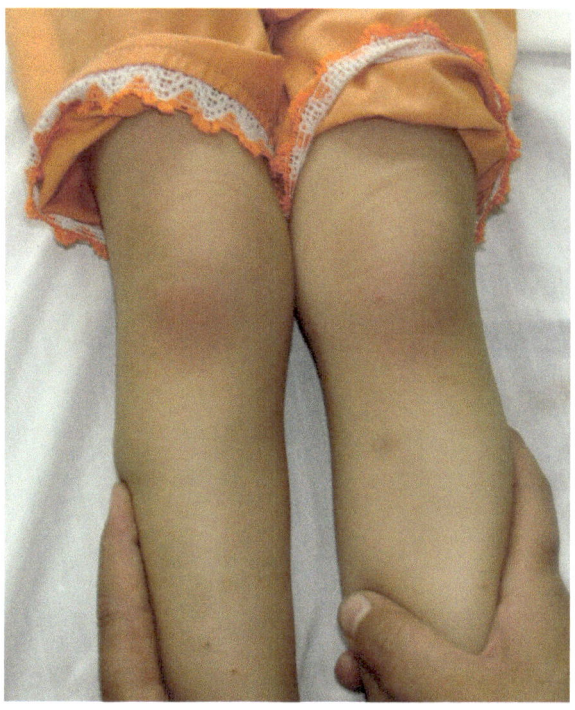

FIGURE 12.4 After treatment (healing of lesions on knee) (Source: Dr. P. Khan Mohammad Beigi, M.D.)

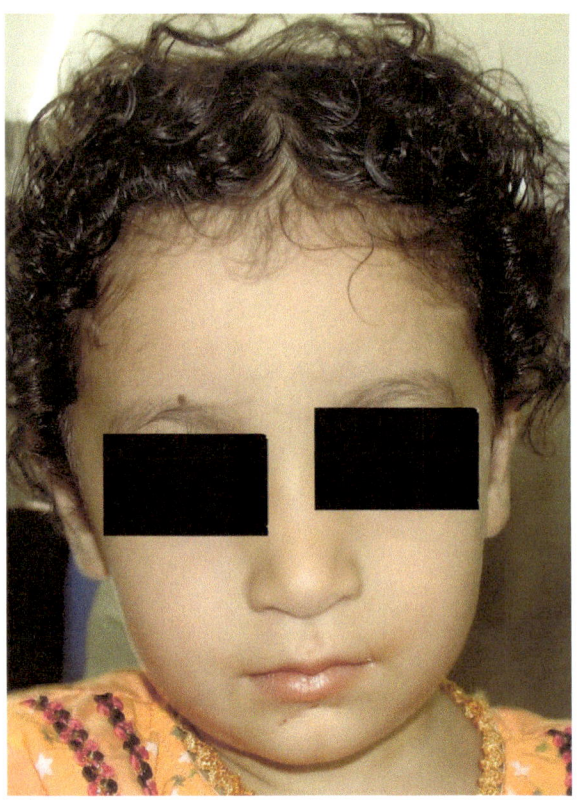

FIGURE 12.5 After treatment (healing of perioral lesions) (Source: Dr. P. Khan Mohammad Beigi, M.D.)

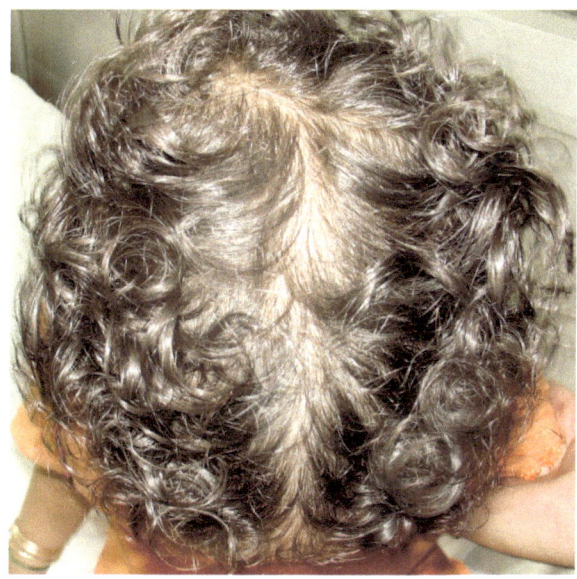

FIGURE 12.6 Hair growth after treatment in a 4-year-old girl (Source: Dr. P. Khan Mohammad Beigi, M.D.)

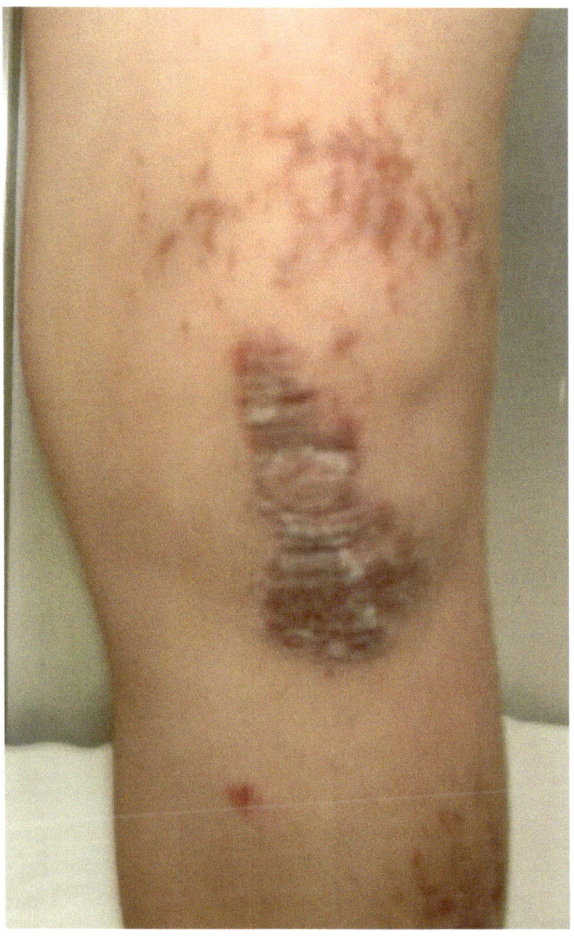

FIGURE 12.7 Psoriasiform plaques with thick yellowish crust on knee
(Source: Dr. P. Khan Mohammad Beigi, M.D.)

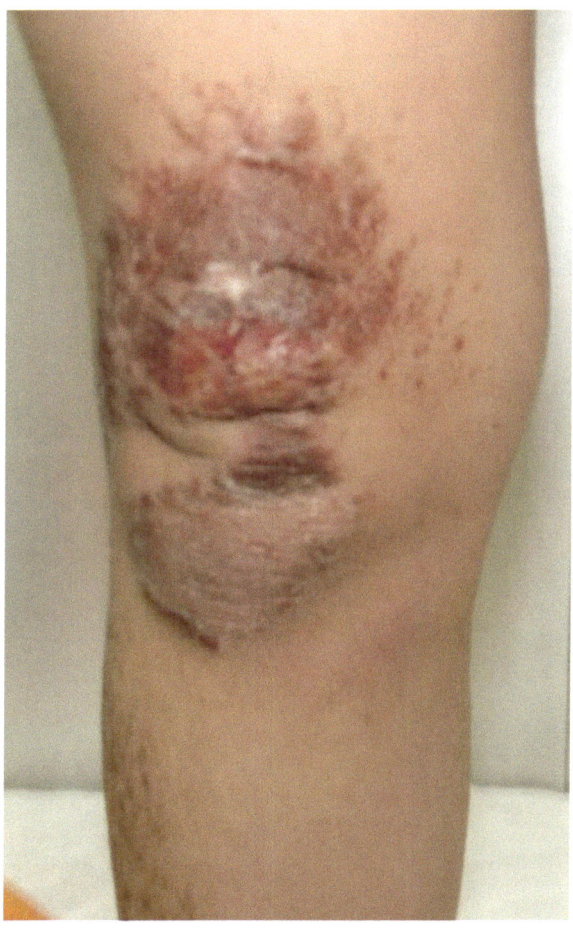

FIGURE 12.8 Crusted eczematoid plaques on knee of 4-year-old boy (Source: Dr. P. Khan Mohammad Beigi, M.D.)

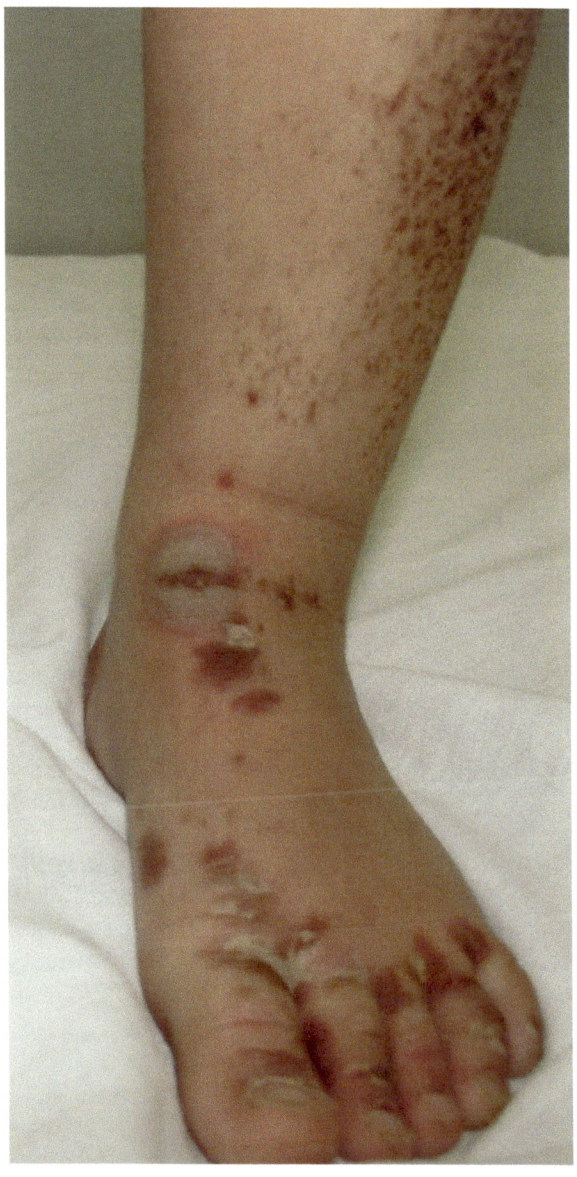

FIGURE 12.9 Discrete crusted lesions on foot and leg of a 4-year-old boy (Source: Dr. P. Khan Mohammad Beigi, M.D.)

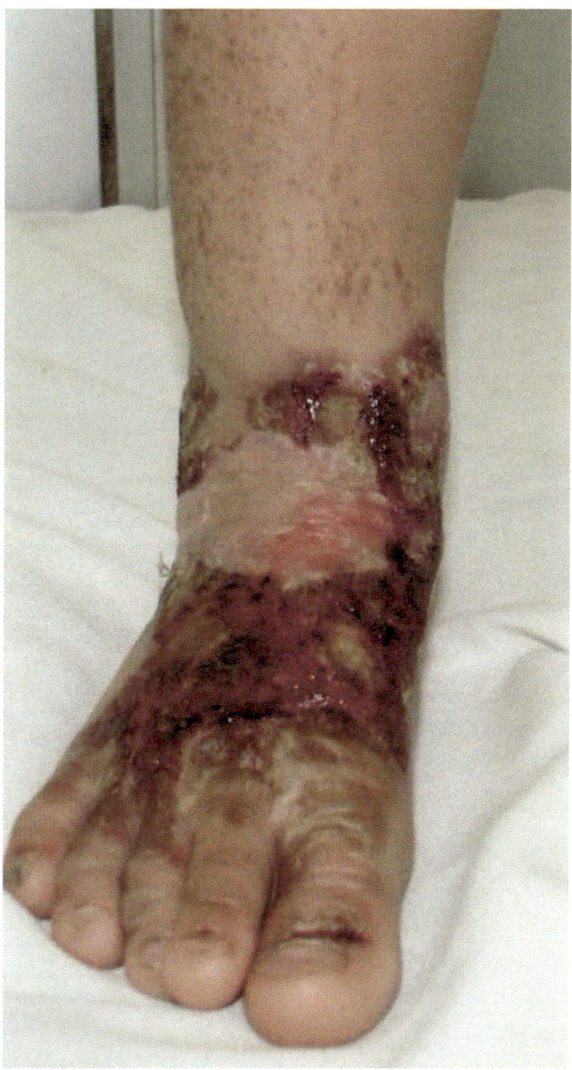

FIGURE 12.10 Erythematous scaling plaques with thick crust on foot and leg of a 4-year-old boy (Source: Dr. P. Khan Mohammad Beigi, M.D.)

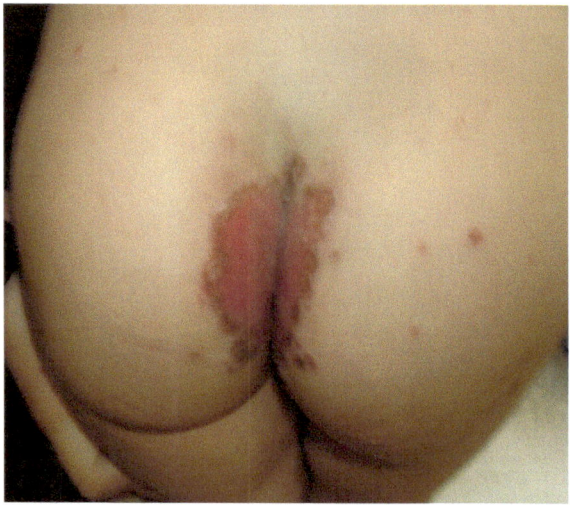

FIGURE 12.11 Perianal crusted oozing patch in a 3-year-old girl (Source: Dr. P. Khan Mohammad Beigi, M.D.)

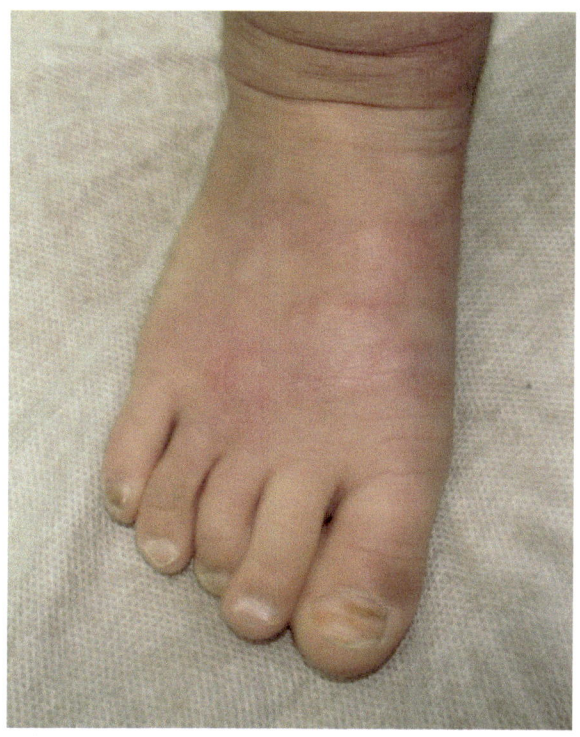

FIGURE 12.12 After treatment (healing of lesions) in a 3-year-old girl (Source: Dr. P. Khan Mohammad Beigi, M.D.)

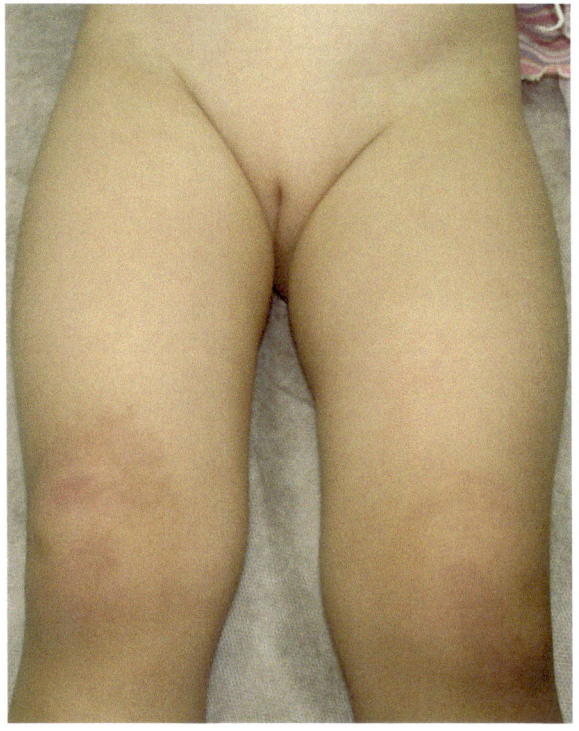

FIGURE 12.13 Healing of lesions on knees after treatment of a 3-year-old girl (Source: Dr. P. Khan Mohammad Beigi, M.D.)

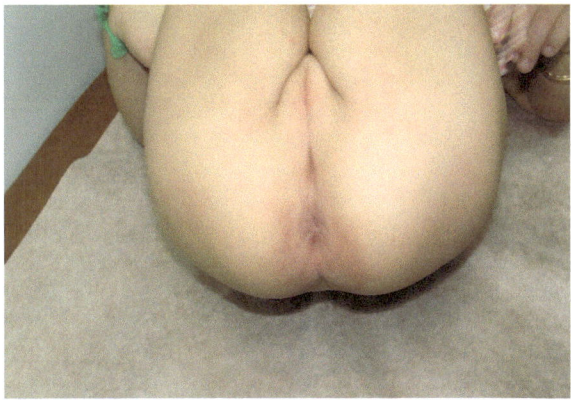

FIGURE 12.14 Healing of perianal lesions after treatment in a 3-year-old girl (Source: Dr. P. Khan Mohammad Beigi, M.D.)

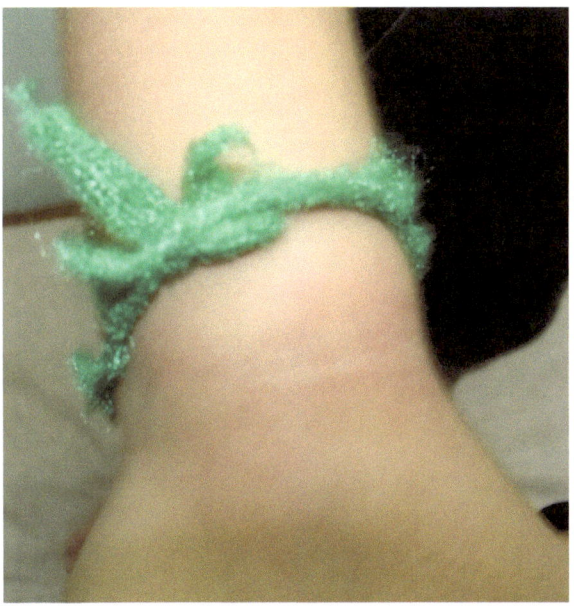

FIGURE 12.15 Healing of lesions after treatment of a 3-year-old girl (Source: Dr. P. Khan Mohammad Beigi, M.D.)

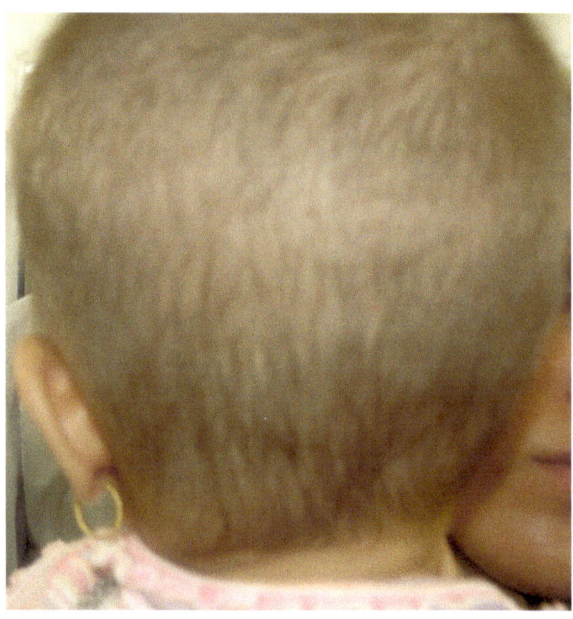

FIGURE 12.16 Partial alopecia with thinning of hair in a 2-year-old girl (Source: Dr. P. Khan Mohammad Beigi, M.D.)

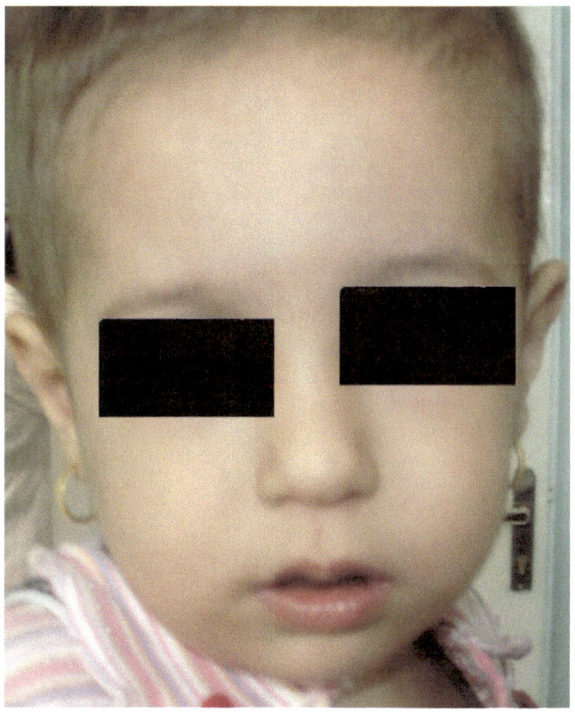

FIGURE 12.17 After treatment (healing of lesions) (Source: Dr. P. Khan Mohammad Beigi, M.D.)

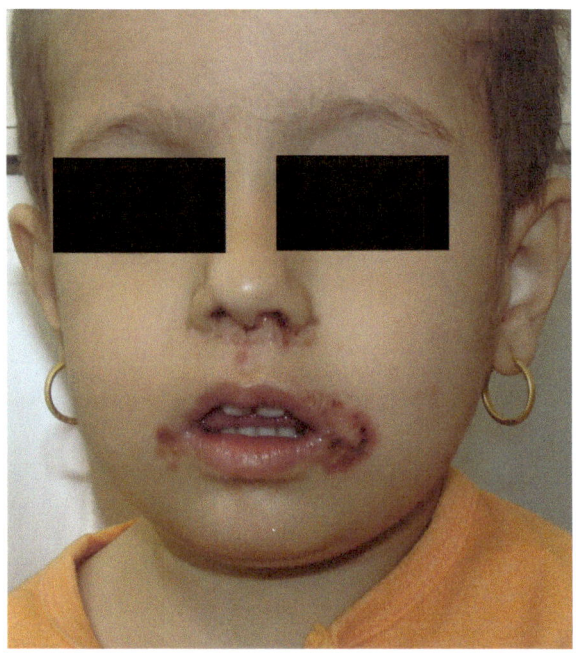

FIGURE 12.18 Perinasal and Perioral Lesions (Source: Dr. P. Khan Mohammad Beigi, M.D.)

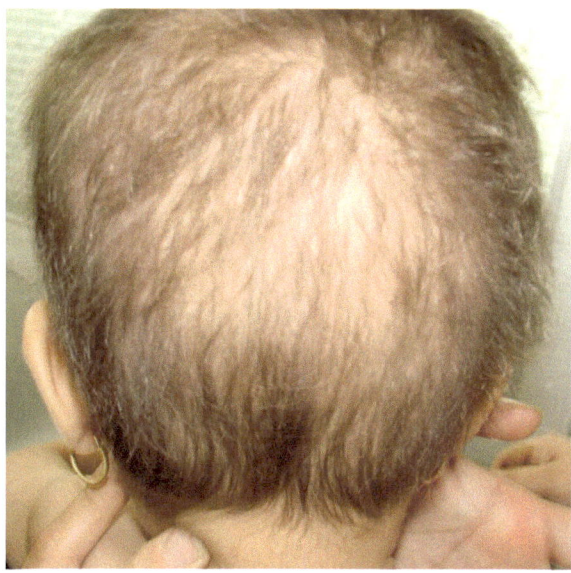

FIGURE 12.19 Presence of Alopecia (Source: Dr. P. Khan Mohammad Beigi, M.D.)

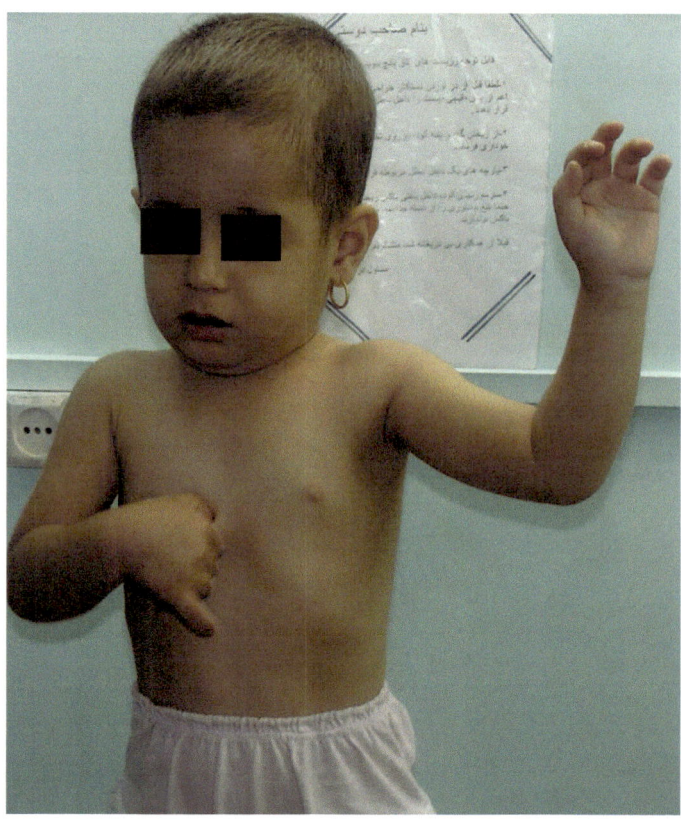

FIGURE 12.20 After treatment (healing of lesions) (Source: Dr. P. Khan Mohammad Beigi, M.D.)

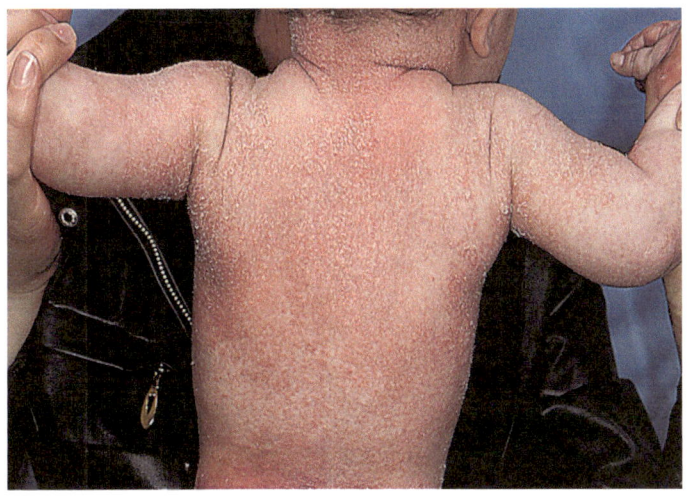

Figure 12.21 Widespread erythematous squamous lesions on trunk and extremities (Source: Dr. P. Khan Mohammad Beigi, M.D.)

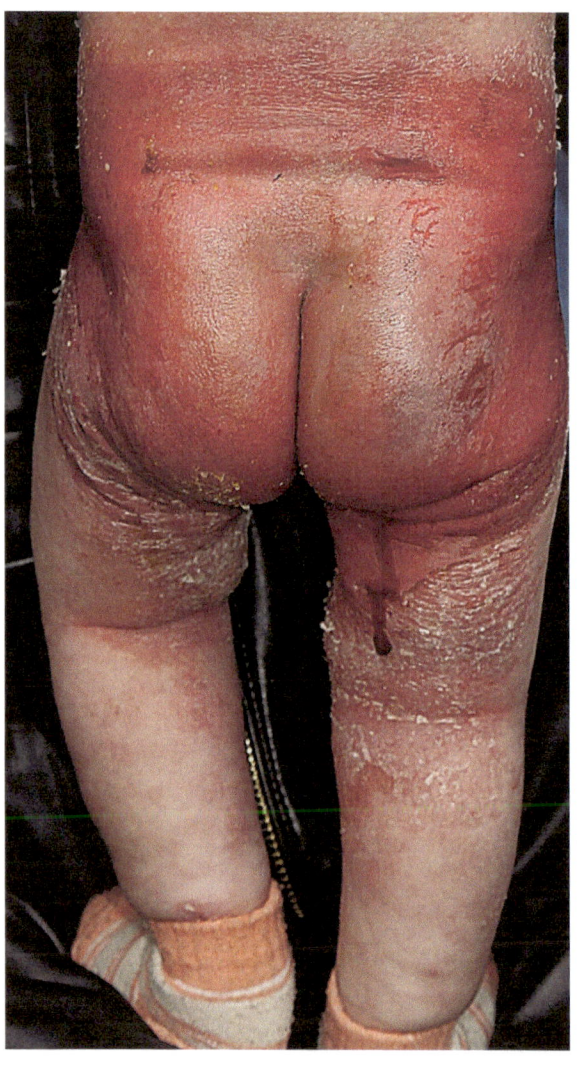

FIGURE 12.22 Widespread erythematous squamous scaly plaques with thick crust on trunk and lower extremities (Source: Dr. P. Khan Mohammad Beigi, M.D.)

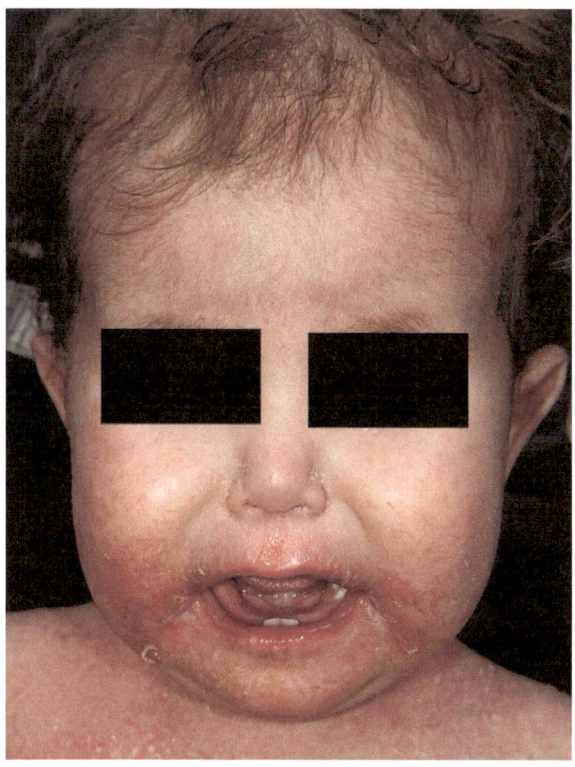

FIGURE 12.23 Perioral lesions in a 3-year-old boy (Source: Dr. P. Khan Mohammad Beigi, M.D.)

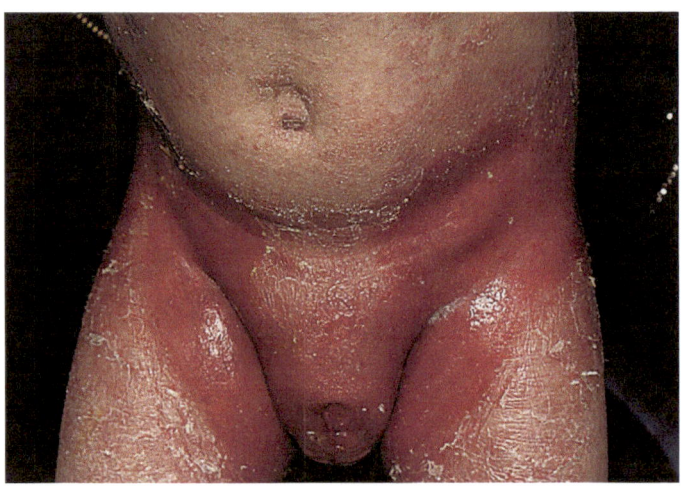

FIGURE 12.24 Oozing lesions on diaper area (Source: Dr. P. Khan Mohammad Beigi, M.D.)

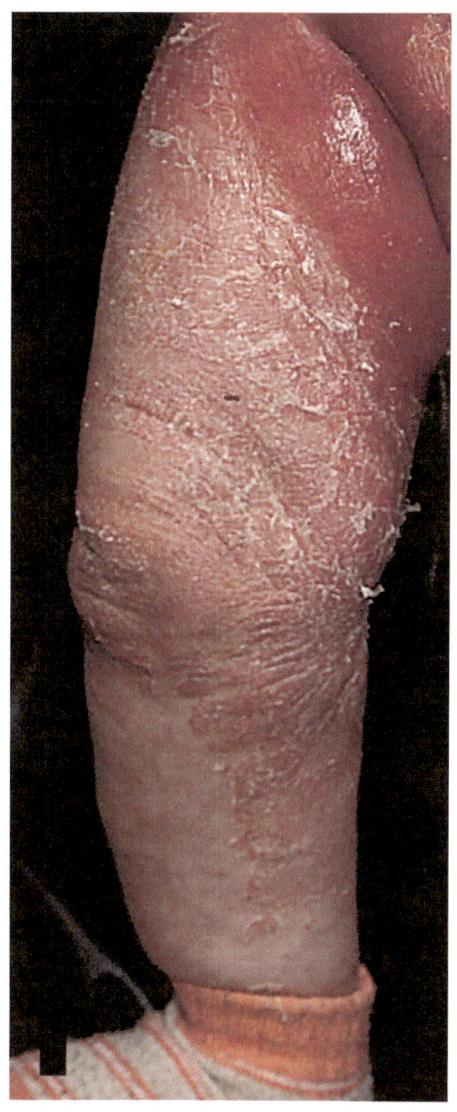

FIGURE 12.25 Crusted scaly lesions on lower extremities of a 1-year-old boy (Source: Dr. P. Khan Mohammad Beigi, M.D.)

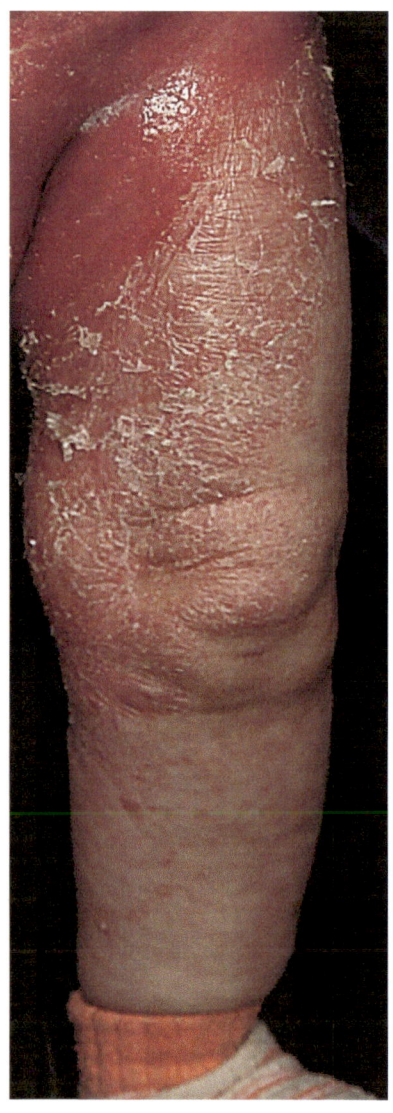

FIGURE 12.26 Crusted scaly lesions on lower extremities of a 1-year-old boy (Source: Dr. P. Khan Mohammad Beigi, M.D.)

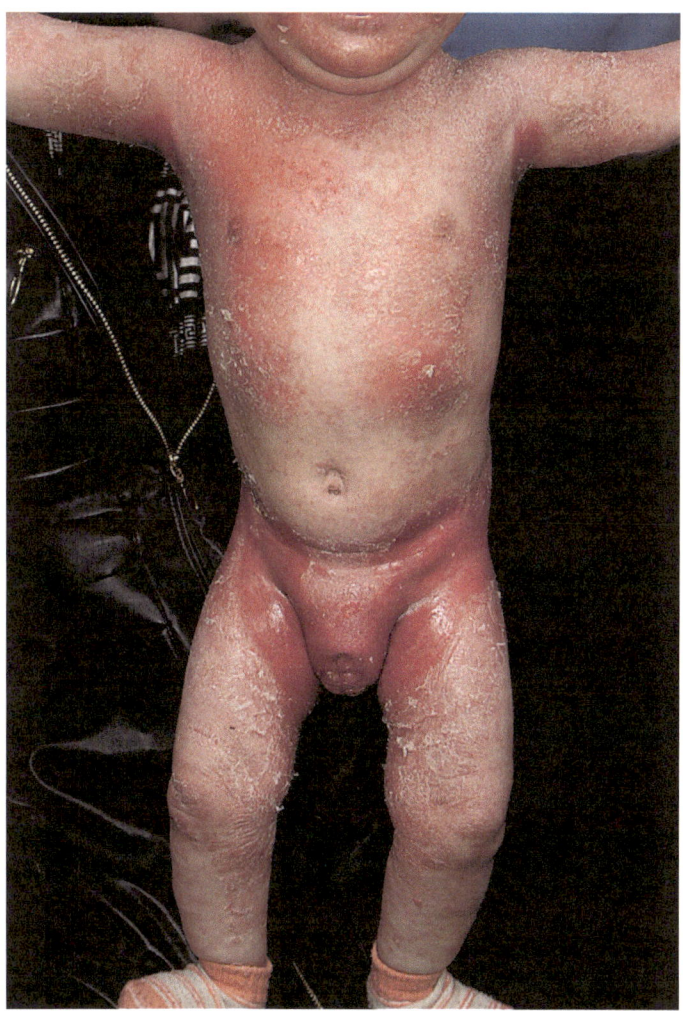

Figure 12.27 Crusted scaly lesions on lower extremities of a 1-year-old boy (Source: Dr. P. Khan Mohammad Beigi, M.D.)

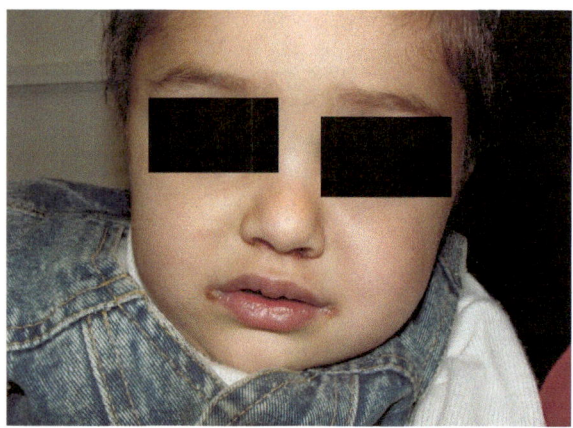

Figure 12.28 Perioral lesions in a 3-year-old boy (Source: Dr. P. Khan Mohammad Beigi, M.D.)

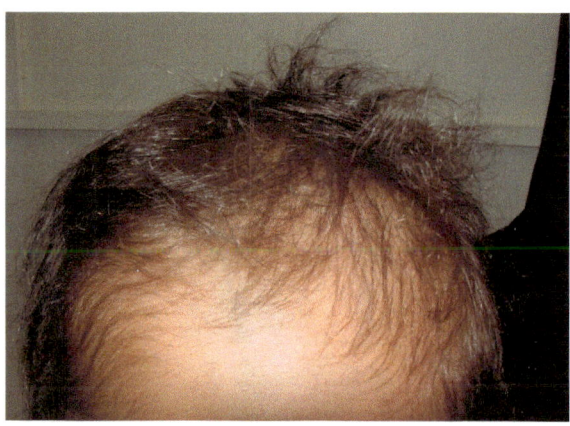

Figure 12.29 Partial alopecia (Source: Dr. P. Khan Mohammad Beigi, M.D.)

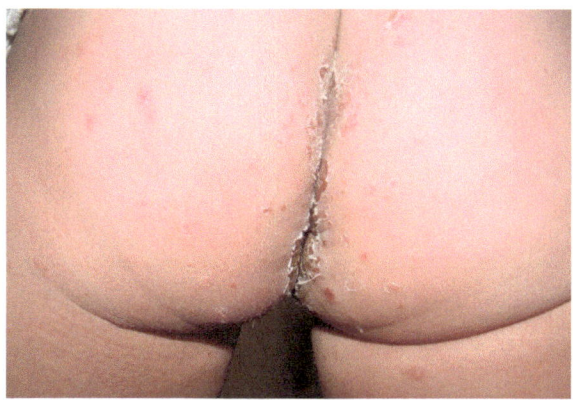

FIGURE 12.30 Crusted perianal lesions (Source: Dr. P. Khan Mohammad Beigi, M.D.)

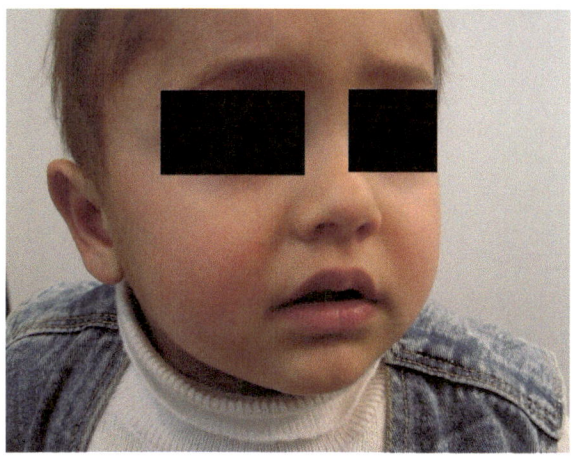

FIGURE 12.31 After treatment (healing of perioral lesions) (Source: Dr. P. Khan Mohammad Beigi, M.D.)

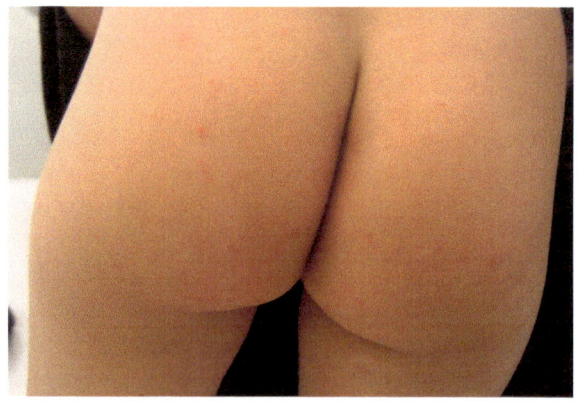

FIGURE 12.32 After treatment (healing of lesions) (Source: Dr. P. Khan Mohammad Beigi, M.D.)

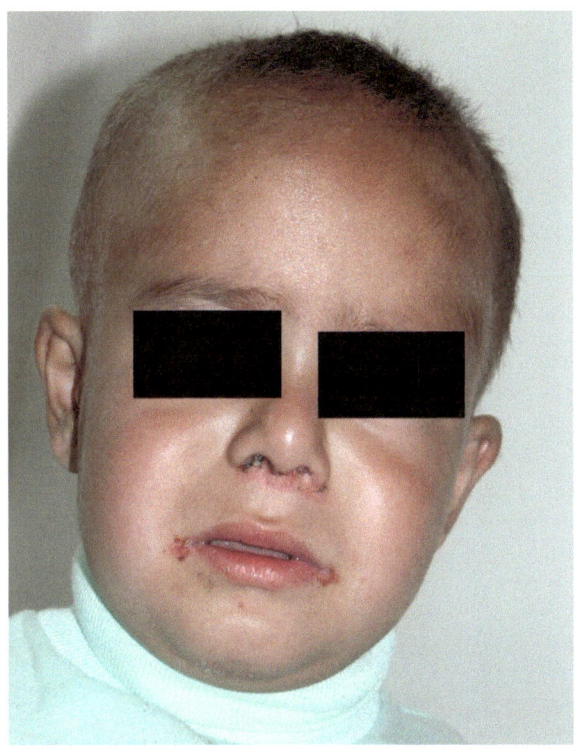

FIGURE 12.33 Periorificial erythematous scaly crusted lesions (Source: Dr. P. Khan Mohammad Beigi, M.D.)

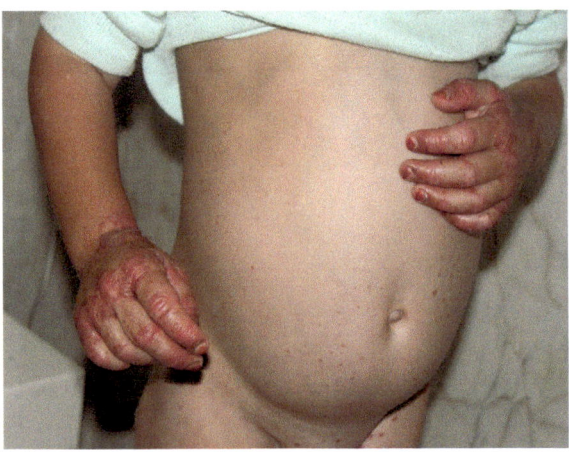

FIGURE 12.34 Oozing crusted erythematous lesions on upper extremities of a 3-year-old boy (Source: Dr. P. Khan Mohammad Beigi, M.D.)

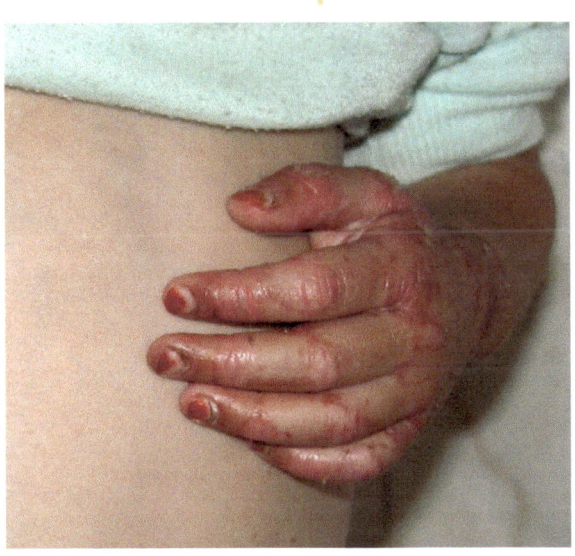

FIGURE 12.35 Oozing crusted erythematous lesions on left hand of a 3-year-old boy (Source: Dr. P. Khan Mohammad Beigi, M.D.)

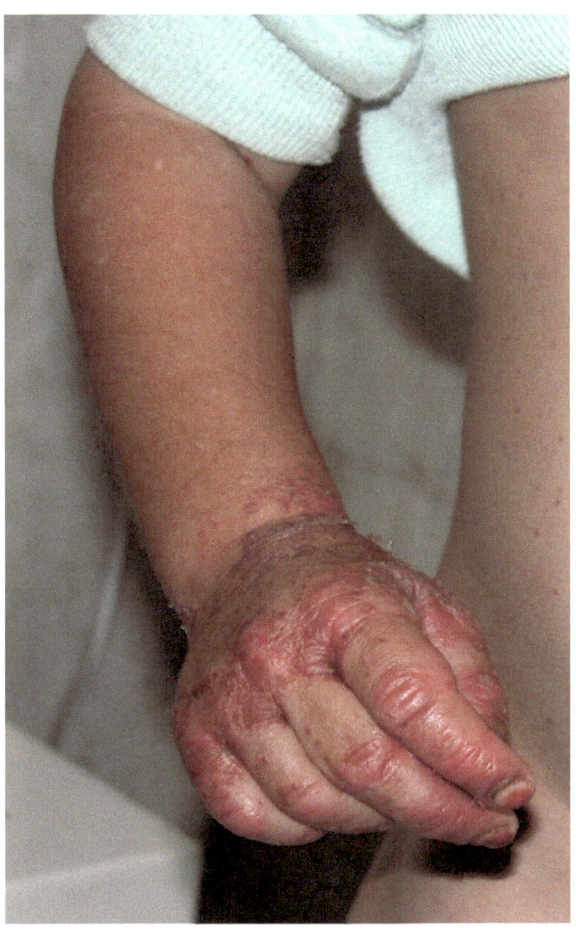

FIGURE 12.36 Oozing crusted erythematous lesions on right hand of a 3-year-old boy (Source: Dr. P. Khan Mohammad Beigi, M.D.)

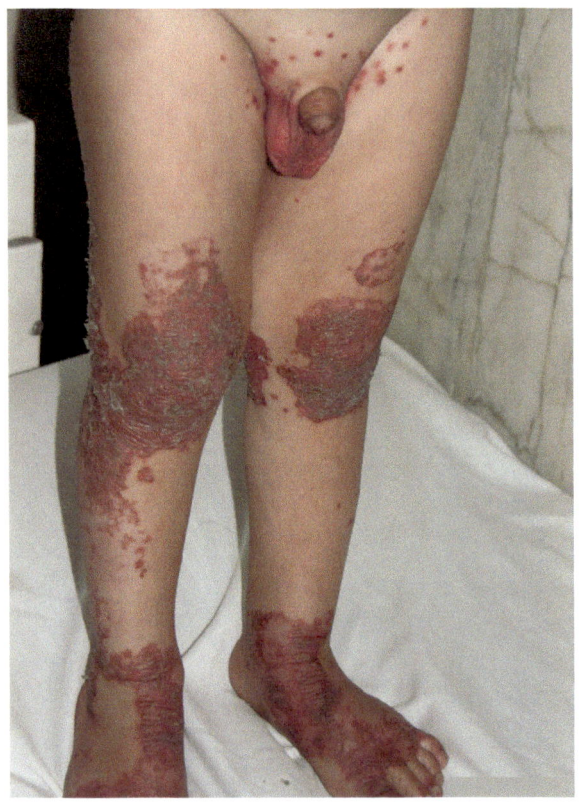

FIGURE 12.37 Crusted eczematoid scaly lesions on lower extremities in a 3-year-old boy (Source: Dr. P. Khan Mohammad Beigi, M.D.)

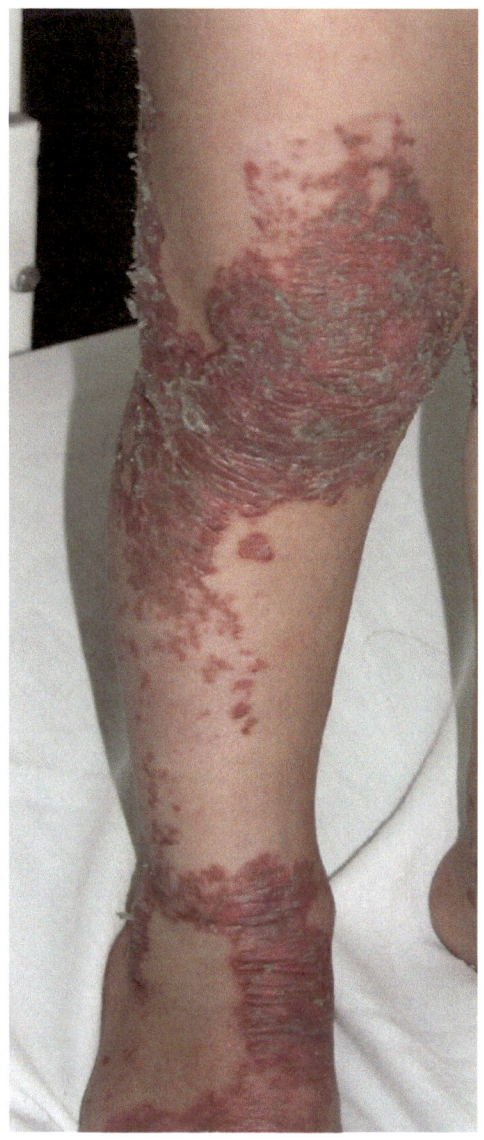

FIGURE 12.38 Crusted eczematoid scaly lesions on lower extremities in a 3-year-old boy (Source: Dr. P. Khan Mohammad Beigi, M.D.)

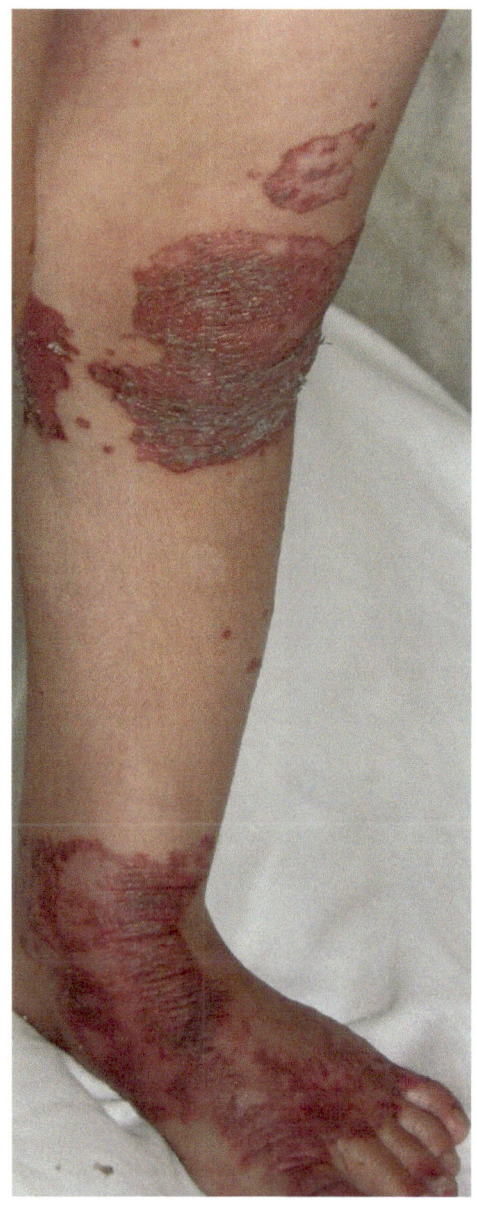

FIGURE 12.39 Eczematoid crusted lesions on knee and foot of a 3-year-old boy (Source: Dr. P. Khan Mohammad Beigi, M.D.)

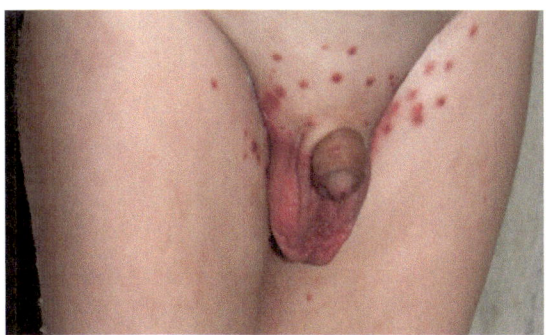

FIGURE 12.40 Lesions on diaper area (Source: Dr. P. Khan Mohammad Beigi, M.D.)

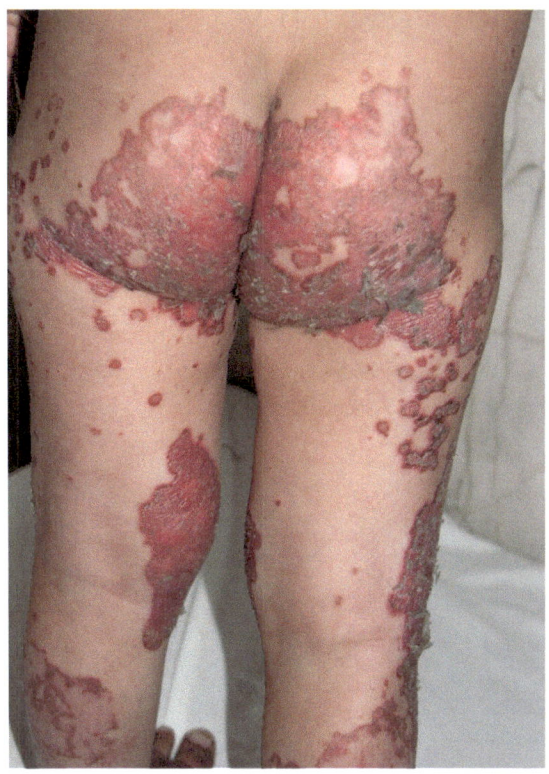

FIGURE 12.41 Eczematoid dermatitis with brownish thick-scaled crust on lower extremities (Source: Dr. P. Khan Mohammad Beigi, M.D.)

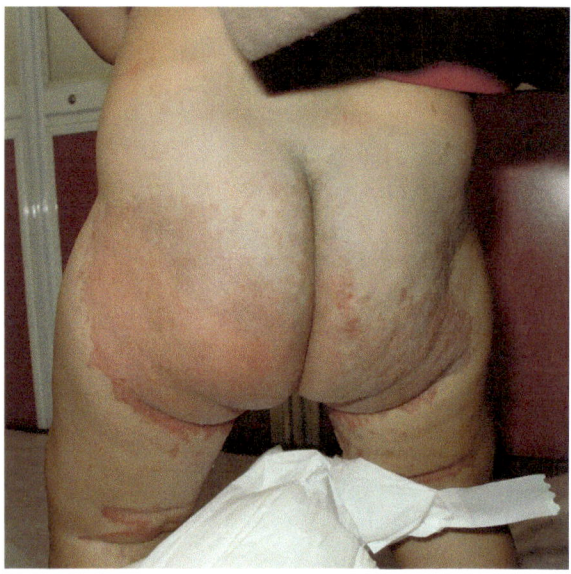

FIGURE 12.42 Eczematoid patches on buttocks and diaper region (Source: Dr. P. Khan Mohammad Beigi, M.D.)

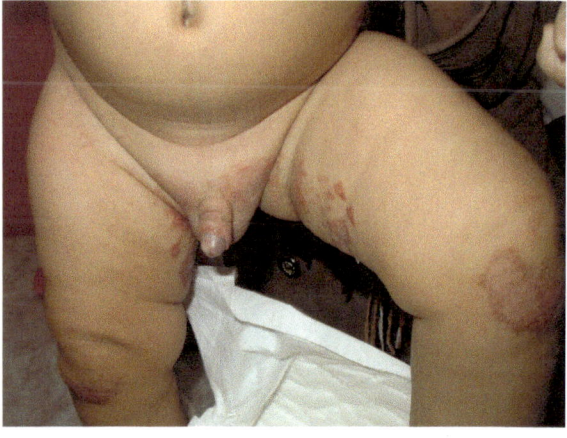

FIGURE 12.43 Erythematous oozing crusted lesions in diaper area of a 2-year-old boy (Source: Dr. P. Khan Mohammad Beigi, M.D.)

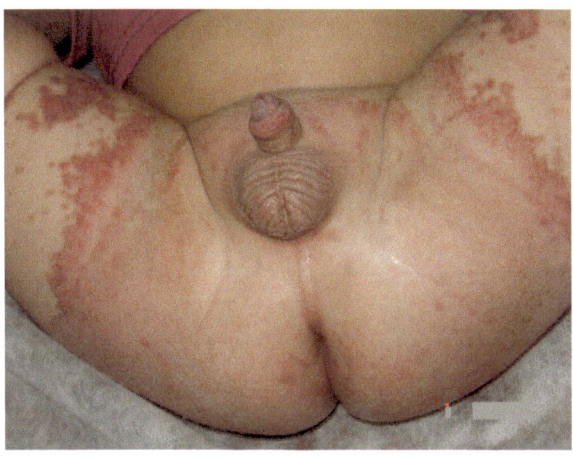

FIGURE 12.44 Erythematous scaly lesions in diaper area of a 2-year-old boy (Source: Dr. P. Khan Mohammad Beigi, M.D.)

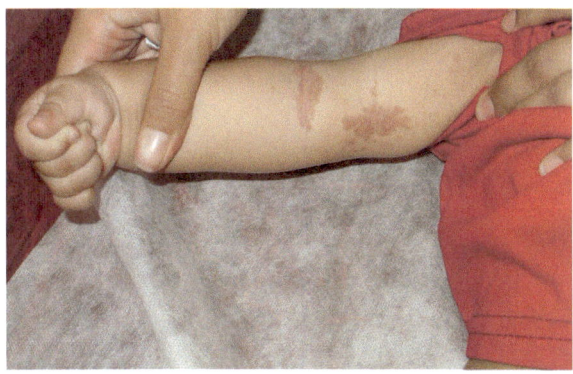

FIGURE 12.45 Psoriasiform and eczematoid lesions of right hand of a 3-year-old girl (Source: Dr. P. Khan Mohammad Beigi, M.D.)

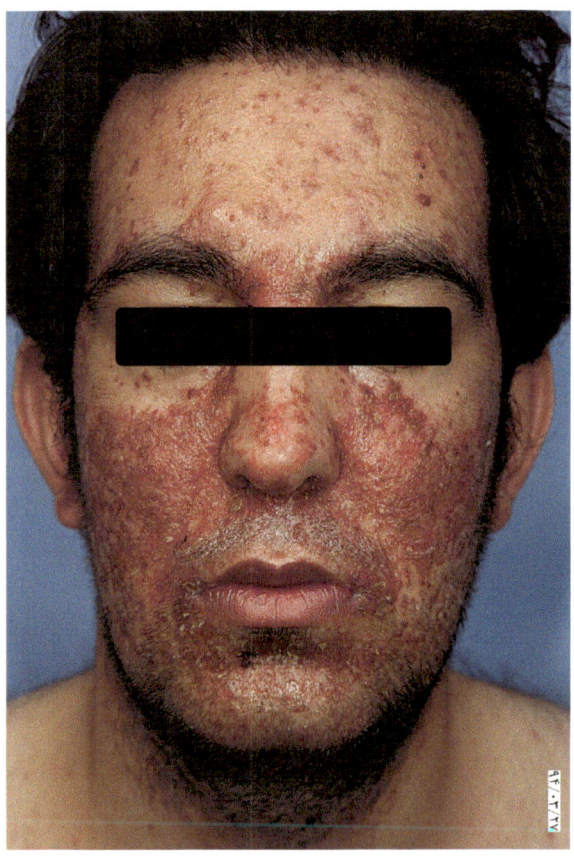

FIGURE 12.46 Recurrence of peri-oral and facial, scaly and papular lesions in a 24-year-old man with a history of zinc deficiency from childhood (Source: Dr. P. Khan Mohammad Beigi, M.D.)

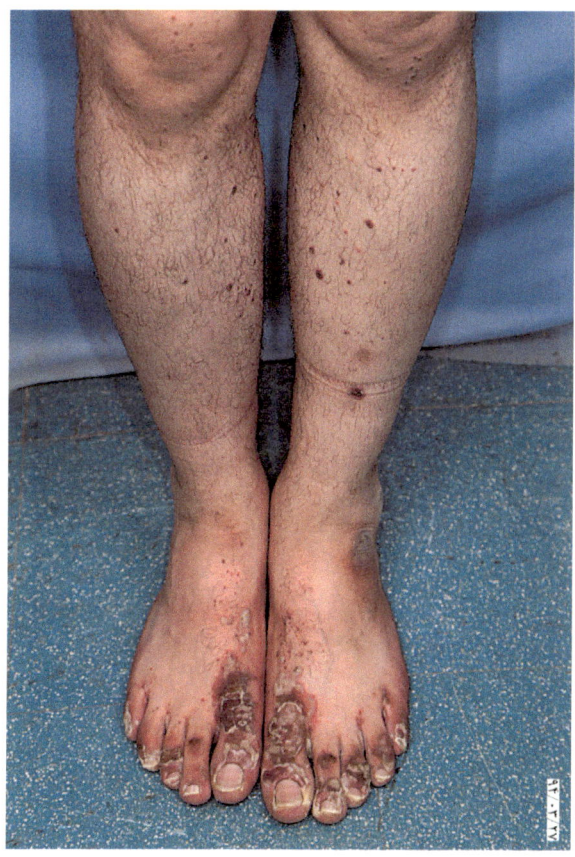

FIGURE 12.47 Erythematous scaling plaques with thick crusts on the lower extremities of a 24-year-old man with a history of zinc deficiency from childhood (Source: Dr. P. Khan Mohammad Beigi, M.D.)

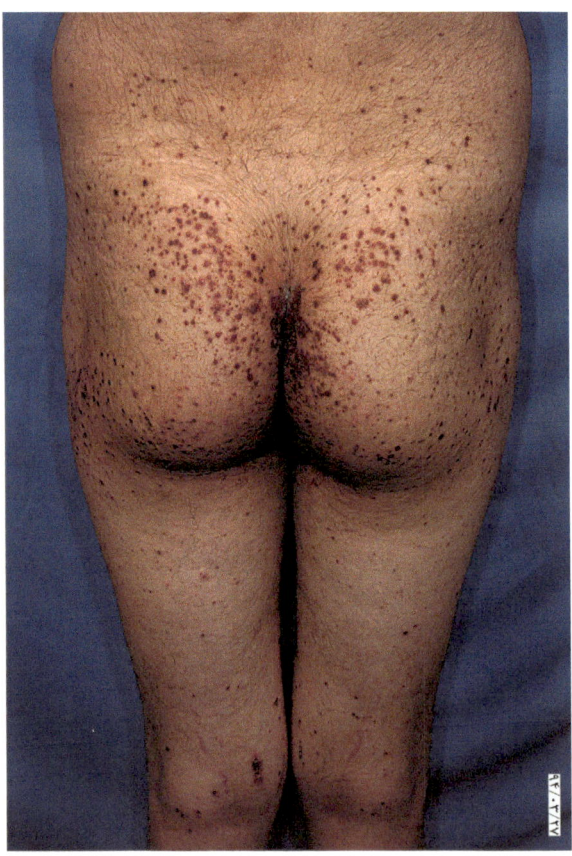

FIGURE 12.48 Recurrence of peri-anal and lower extremities papular lesions in a 24-year-old man with a history of zinc deficiency (Source: Dr. P. Khan Mohammad Beigi, M.D.)

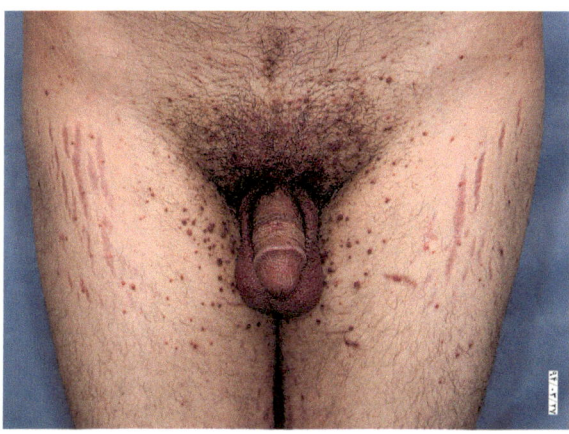

FIGURE 12.49 Recurrence of perineal and peri-genital lesions in a 24-year-old man with a history of zinc deficiency (Source: Dr. P. Khan Mohammad Beigi, M.D.)

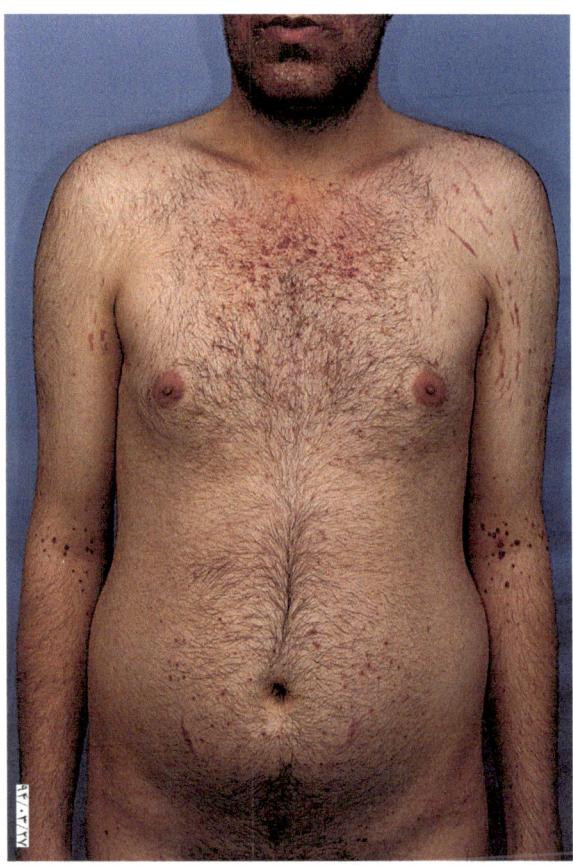

FIGURE 12.50 Recurrence of erythematous papular lesions in a 24-year-old man with a history of zinc deficiency (Source: Dr. P. Khan Mohammad Beigi, M.D.)

Index

P. Khan Mohammad Beigi, E. Maverakis,   155
Acrodermatitis Enteropathica: A Clinician's Guide,
DOI 10.1007/978-3-319-17819-6,
© Springer International Publishing Switzerland 2015